KU-014-636

Contents

Acknowledgements   v

Introduction   1

Chapter 1. Health and the urban crisis   5
Urban growth   5
Urbanization policies in developing countries   21
The urban poor   25
Health consequences of rapid urban growth   29
Distinctive characteristics of urban poverty   43
Comprehensive coverage   45

Chapter 2. Reorienting urban health systems   46
The primary health care approach   48
Applying the primary health care approach
   in the cities   53
Equity   54
Assessing the state of health in urban areas   56
Health systems research   63
Priorities in introducing primary health care   66
Resources: money, people, and imagination   69
Orientation, education, and training   71
Financing primary health care in urban areas   75
Urban health departments   77
Hospitals: the untapped resource   80
Implementation   83
Managing urban change   84

Chapter 3. Community involvement   88
Linking health systems and communities   88
Local organizations for community involvement   91
The role of facilitators   97
Community health workers   100
Examples of community involvement   107
Support to enable communities to help
     themselves   108
Communities and financing   110

**Chapter 4. Health and health-related development
      in urban areas**   112
Socioeconomic development and health   112
Intersectoral coordination in urban areas   112
Urban development   119
Employment, income, and nutrition   123
Low-income housing   126
Legislation and legalization   127
Water supply and sanitation   128
Literacy and education   134
Multisectoral projects with a health component   137

Chapter 5. Towards universal coverage   141
Health for all: responsibility of all   141
National strategies for urban health systems   142
Strengthening ministries of health for primary
     health care   143
From projects to major programmes   144
Collaboration between governments and
     nongovernmental organizations   151
Collaboration between cities   154

Chapter 6. Conclusions   156
References   158
**Annex. Indicators of social development in
     Thailand**   166

SPOTLIGHT ON THE CITIES

Improving urban health in developing countries

I. Tabibzadeh

Responsible Medical Officer,
National Health
Systems and Policies,
Division of
Strengthening of
Health Services,
World Health
Organization,
Geneva, Switzerland

A. Rossi-Espagnet

Former Chief Medical
Officer,
Division of
Strengthening of
Health Services,
World Health
Organization,
Geneva, Switzerland

and

R. Maxwell

Secretary,
King Edward's Hospital
Fund for London,
London, England

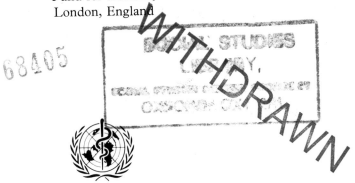

World Health Organization
Geneva 1989

WHO Library Cataloguing in Publication Data

Tabibzadeh, I.
    Spotlight on the cities : improving urban health in developing countries.

    1.Urban health   2.Urban population   3.Delivery of health care
    4.Developing countries   I.Rossi-Espagnet, A.   II.Maxwell, R.
    III.Title

    ISBN 92 4 156131 9   (NLM Classification: WA 380)

© World Health Organization 1989

TYPESET IN INDIA
PRINTED IN ENGLAND
89/7937–Macmillan/Clays–8000

Acknowledgements

This publication is a review, synthesis, and elaboration of the following unpublished WHO documents: *Primary health care in urban areas: reaching the urban poor in developing countries*, prepared by UNICEF and WHO (document SHS/84.4); *Joint UNICEF/WHO Consultation on Primary Health Care in Urban Areas, Guayaquil, Ecuador* (document SHS/84.5); and *UNICEF/WHO Interregional Consultation on Primary Health Care in Urban Areas, Manila, Philippines, 7–11 July 1986*. The demographic data contained in these documents have been updated as required.

Numerous national and international officers contributed to these reports. We thank the national participants in the above consultations, and are grateful in particular for the contributions made by: Mr W. J. Cousins, UNICEF; Mr J. H. Donohue, UNICEF; Dr T. Harpham, London School of Hygiene and Tropical Medicine, England; Dr S. Rifkin, Liverpool School of Tropical Medicine, England; Mr C. Shubert, UNICEF; and Dr G. Stott, Geneva, Switzerland. In addition, we are grateful to the following staff at WHO headquarters for their comments and contributions to this publication: Mr M. A. Acheson, Mr A. Creese, Mr G. Goldstein, Mr J. M. Jackson, Dr H. M. Kahssay, Dr. S. Khanna, Dr S. Litsios, Mr A. D. Lopez, Mr R. Novick, Dr P. M. Shah, and Dr D. Smith. Thanks are also due to Miss B. Pumfrey for help with the illustrations and to Mrs C. Riley for secretarial assistance. Finally, we thank Professor V. Ramalingaswami, Adviser to the Executive Director, UNICEF, and Professor C. Taylor, School of Hygiene and Public Health, Johns Hopkins University, Baltimore, MD, USA.

The photograph on page 31 was a winning entry in the UN photo competition, "A better way to live".

Introduction

This publication is about the health of the poor in the fast-expanding cities of the poorer countries of the world. The subject is immensely important, fascinating, and verging on tragedy. Yet until recently it was largely ignored. Most people were simply unaware of the gravity of the situation. For city and national governments already facing tough challenges, and with little money, there is no incentive to search for undiagnosed difficulties, until they simply cannot be ignored any more. The facts themselves are frequently unknown because so often the poorest communities in the cities concerned are unmapped in a statistical sense and lack official recognition; when demographic data and morbidity statistics are collected, those for poorer areas tend to be grossly under-recorded and are quickly lost in city averages, diluted by the returns from more prosperous neighbourhoods. At times there seems to be a conspiracy of silence about health in urban districts, particularly those that are unserved or underserved.

But the story is not without hope. It is full of human interest, testifying as it does to a quiet, unselfish courage, particularly among women bringing up children in great poverty. Moreover, much help can be provided at modest cost, as many successful local initiatives have proved. The next major hurdle is to apply the lessons of these initiatives much more widely, moving towards universal health coverage in the poorest urban communities. It is not new knowledge that is needed so much as new awareness and the determination to apply what is already known. What is required is inherent in the principles of primary health care. Indeed the Declaration of Alma-Ata of September 1978 specifically mentions urban as well as rural development (*1*). Similarly the WHO Global Strategy for Health for All by the Year 2000 refers explicitly to urbanization and its attendant problems (*2*). If many people in the World Health Organization and elsewhere saw rural poverty as the top priority in the early 1980s, nobody should ignore the equally urgent (and in

1

some respects sharply different) problems of urban poverty in the 1990s.

The aims of this publication, therefore, are to:

- alert people to the scale, nature, urgency, and near desperation of the predicament of the poor in many cities of the world;

- advocate a fundamental shift in health care priorities and strategies in the cities, from simply trying to do more of the same to applying primary health care principles in practice. This is a message not only for ministries of health, but equally for city hospitals and medical schools, the medical profession, city health departments, and political leaders at the city and national levels;

- explain some of the key characteristics of successful action to improve urban health, as reflected in actual local experience: for example the indispensable elements of community involvement and intersectoral action;

- focus attention upon the urgent need to raise one's sights from successful pockets of action to comprehensive coverage: unless this is done (and done quickly) there is simply no hope of action on an adequate scale.

Government plans and programmes must be prospectively oriented—in other words, based not only on a good knowledge of prevailing conditions and problems, but also on the way they are expected to evolve in the future. Thus, Chapter 1 gives some facts, figures, and trends related to urbanization. These speak for themselves, but "numbers do not tell the whole story and no amount of statistics or reports can convey the true feeling and the real dimension of the destitution and even abjectness under which large populations in many cities of the world are forced to live. Only exposure to that destitution and direct observation of it can create the awareness and motivation required for dedicated involvement" (3).

Hence, this publication is addressed to a wide range of political leaders and managers responsible for the health and social welfare of low-income, underserved urban populations; health workers at different levels; city planners; and international and nongovernmental organizations and funding agencies concerned with the problems of the urban poor in developing countries.

Preparing a document for publication is usually harder than one expects, and there is always satisfaction in its completion. But no other publication we have been involved with has left us with quite

2

the same feelings about the urgency of its message, or the same sense of the privilege of being associated with a human endeavour of the highest importance. The urban poor not only need help, they have the right to ask it from all of us, and they must not ask in vain.

Chapter 1

Health and the urban crisis

Throughout the 1960s and 1970s, the main emphasis in community health in developing countries was on extending health service coverage in the rural areas, hitherto largely unserved but containing 85% of the population. During that period, relatively little attention was paid to the urban situation, which was fast deteriorating with the continued migration of people to the towns (*4*).

However, since the beginning of the 1980s, authorities throughout the world have become increasingly concerned with the great public health problems found in the cities.

The 1980 Rome Declaration on Population and the Urban Future (*5,6*) pointed out that "in the next two decades, the world will undergo, as a result of the urbanization process, the most radical changes ever in social, economic and political life". However, far from constituting an indication of social development and of economic and cultural progress, the chaotic, unbalanced and uncontrolled growth of urban centres has become a source of major concern for political leaders, social planners, and administrators, especially in the developing world. The Rome Declaration therefore castigated the inadequacies, in most cities of the world, of "virtually every service amenity and support required for tolerable urban living".

Urban growth

The world population is expected to reach 6122 million by the year 2000 and 8206 million by 2025 (Table 1), an increase of 26% between 1985 and 2000 and a further 34% between 2000 and 2025.[1]

---

[1] Unless otherwise noted, all figures in this section are based on the projections prepared by the United Nations Department of International Economic and Social Affairs.

Table 1. Estimated and projected total, urban, and rural population, by region or area, 1970–2025 (millions)[a]

Region or area		1970	1975	1980	1985	1990	1995	2000	2005	2010	2015	2020	2025
World total	total	3 693	4 076	4 450	4 837	5 246	5 678	6 122	6 559	6 989	7 414	7 822	8 206
	urban	1 371	1 564	1 764	1 983	2 234	2 525	2 854	3 220	3 623	4 050	4 488	4 932
	rural	2 322	2 512	2 685	2 854	3 012	3 153	3 268	3 339	3 366	3 364	3 334	3 274
Developed regions	total	1 047	1 095	1 137	1 174	1 210	1 244	1 277	1 305	1 331	1 355	1 377	1 396
	urban	698	753	798	839	877	915	950	983	1 011	1 039	1 063	1 087
	rural	350	341	338	335	333	329	327	323	320	316	313	310
Developing regions	total	2 646	2 981	3 313	3 663	4 036	4 434	4 845	5 254	5 658	6 059	6 446	6 809
	urban	673	811	966	1 144	1 357	1 610	1 904	2 237	2 612	3 011	3 425	3 845
	rural	1 973	2 171	2 347	2 519	2 679	2 824	2 941	3 016	3 046	3 048	3 021	2 964
Africa	total	361	413	479	555	645	751	872	1 008	1 158	1 313	1 468	1 617
	urban	81	101	129	165	210	268	340	426	528	642	766	894
	rural	280	312	350	390	435	482	532	582	630	671	702	722
Eastern Africa	total	106	122	143	166	196	231	272	320	373	429	484	537
	urban	11	15	21	30	42	57	77	102	133	168	206	246
	rural	95	107	121	136	154	173	195	218	240	261	278	291
Middle Africa	total	40	45	52	60	69	79	92	106	122	138	154	170
	urban	10	13	16	21	27	35	44	55	67	81	95	110
	rural	30	33	36	38	41	45	48	52	55	57	59	60
Northern Africa	total	83	94	108	123	140	158	176	193	211	228	245	261
	urban	30	36	43	52	62	75	89	104	120	137	154	172
	rural	53	58	65	71	78	83	87	89	91	91	90	89
Southern Africa	total	26	29	33	37	42	48	55	61	69	76	84	91
	urban	11	14	16	20	23	28	33	39	45	52	60	67
	rural	14	15	17	18	19	20	21	22	23	24	24	24
Western Africa	total	106	123	144	169	199	235	277	327	383	442	501	558
	urban	19	24	32	42	55	73	97	126	163	205	251	300
	rural	87	99	112	127	143	161	181	201	220	237	250	259

Americas	total	510	560	613	668	726	785	844	901	959	1 017	1 072	1 124
	urban	330	374	423	475	530	586	642	699	755	812	868	923
	rural	180	186	191	194	197	199	201	203	204	205	204	201
Latin America	total	283	321	361	405	451	499	546	594	642	689	735	779
	urban	163	198	236	279	325	372	420	467	515	563	610	656
	rural	121	124	125	125	126	126	127	127	127	127	125	123
Caribbean	total	25	27	30	32	35	38	41	44	48	51	55	58
	urban	11	14	16	18	21	24	27	30	33	36	40	43
	rural	13	14	14	14	14	14	14	15	15	15	15	15
Central America	total	68	80	92	105	119	134	149	164	179	194	209	223
	urban	37	46	56	66	79	92	105	119	134	149	163	178
	rural	31	34	36	39	41	42	44	45	45	46	45	45
Temperate South America	total	36	39	42	46	49	52	55	58	61	64	67	70
	urban	28	31	35	38	42	46	49	52	56	59	62	64
	rural	8	8	7	7	7	7	6	6	6	6	5	5
Tropical South America	total	154	175	198	222	248	275	301	327	354	380	405	429
	urban	86	107	130	156	184	211	239	266	293	319	345	370
	rural	68	68	67	66	64	63	62	61	61	60	60	58
Northern America	total	227	239	252	264	275	287	297	307	317	327	337	345
	urban	167	176	186	195	204	214	223	231	240	249	258	267
	rural	59	62	66	68	71	73	75	76	77	78	79	79
Asia	total	2 102	2 354	2 584	2 818	3 058	3 304	3 549	3 775	3 982	4 180	4 365	4 535
	urban	503	595	688	791	915	1 066	1 242	1 444	1 670	1 908	2 151	2 397
	rural	1 599	1 759	1 896	2 027	2 143	2 239	2 306	2 330	2 312	2 272	2 214	2 138

[a] Source: United Nations (7).

7

Table 1. (continued)

Region or area		1970	1975	1980	1985	1990	1995	2000	2005	2010	2015	2020	2025
East Asia	total	986	1 096	1 176	1 250	1 324	1 399	1 475	1 539	1 589	1 634	1 679	1 721
	urban	266	302	331	357	391	433	485	547	618	692	770	849
	rural	721	794	846	892	933	967	990	992	971	942	909	872
China	total	831	927	996	1 060	1 124	1 190	1 256	1 311	1 355	1 396	1 436	1 475
	urban	167	187	203	219	241	272	315	367	431	499	570	645
	rural	664	740	793	841	883	917	941	944	924	897	866	830
Japan	total	104	112	117	121	124	127	130	132	133	133	133	132
	urban	74	84	89	92	95	98	101	103	105	106	106	106
	rural	30	27	28	28	29	29	29	29	28	27	27	26
Other East Asia	total	51	57	63	69	76	83	89	95	101	105	110	114
	urban	24	31	38	46	55	63	70	76	82	88	93	98
	rural	27	27	25	23	22	21	20	19	18	17	17	16
South Asia	total	1 116	1 258	1 408	1 568	1 734	1 905	2 074	2 236	2 394	2 546	2 686	2 814
	urban	237	293	358	434	524	633	757	898	1 052	1 215	1 381	1 548
	rural	879	965	1 050	1 135	1 209	1 272	1 317	1 339	1 341	1 330	1 304	1 266
Southeastern Asia	total	288	324	361	400	439	480	520	557	593	627	659	688
	urban	58	71	87	105	127	154	184	219	256	294	334	374
	rural	230	253	274	295	312	326	335	339	337	333	325	315
Southern Asia	total	754	849	949	1 056	1 165	1 277	1 387	1 491	1 592	1 689	1 777	1 855
	urban	147	181	220	267	322	388	466	553	652	756	863	968
	rural	607	668	728	789	843	889	921	938	940	932	914	886
Western Asia	total	74	85	98	113	130	148	168	188	209	230	250	271
	urban	32	41	51	62	75	91	107	125	145	165	185	205
	rural	42	44	48	51	54	57	60	63	64	65	65	65

Europe	total	459	474	485	492	499	506	512	517	520	521	523	524
	urban	306	326	340	352	363	374	385	393	400	406	412	417
	rural	153	148	144	140	135	131	128	123	119	115	111	107
Eastern Europe	total	103	106	109	112	115	118	120	123	125	127	129	131
	urban	55	60	65	69	73	77	80	84	87	89	92	94
	rural	48	46	44	43	42	41	40	39	38	38	37	37
Northern Europe	total	80	82	82	83	83	83	84	84	84	84	84	84
	urban	66	69	70	71	72	73	74	74	75	75	76	76
	rural	14	13	12	12	11	10	10	9	9	9	8	8
Southern Europe	total	128	134	140	143	146	149	152	155	156	157	158	159
	urban	72	78	84	89	94	99	104	108	112	116	119	122
	rural	56	56	55	54	52	50	49	46	44	42	40	37
Western Europe	total	148	152	154	154	155	156	156	155	154	153	152	150
	urban	113	119	121	123	124	126	127	127	127	126	126	125
	rural	35	33	32	31	31	30	29	28	28	27	26	25
USSR	total	242	253	265	279	292	304	315	326	337	348	358	368
	urban	137	152	167	183	197	211	222	234	245	256	264	273
	rural	105	101	98	96	95	93	92	92	92	93	94	95
Oceania	total	19	21	23	25	26	28	30	32	33	35	36	38
	urban	14	15	16	18	19	20	21	23	24	26	27	29
	rural	6	6	7	7	8	8	9	9	9	9	9	9
Australia/New Zealand	total	15	17	18	19	20	21	22	23	24	25	26	27
	urban	13	14	15	16	17	18	19	20	21	22	23	24
	rural	2	2	3	3	3	3	3	3	3	3	3	3
Melanesia	total	3	4	4	5	5	6	7	7	8	9	9	10
	urban	0	1	1	1	1	1	2	2	3	3	4	4
	rural	3	3	3	4	4	5	5	5	5	6	6	6
Micronesia/Polynesia	total	1	1	1	1	1	1	1	1	1	1	1	1
	urban	0	0	0	0	0	0	1	1	1	1	1	1
	rural	0	0	0	1	1	1	1	1	0	0	0	0

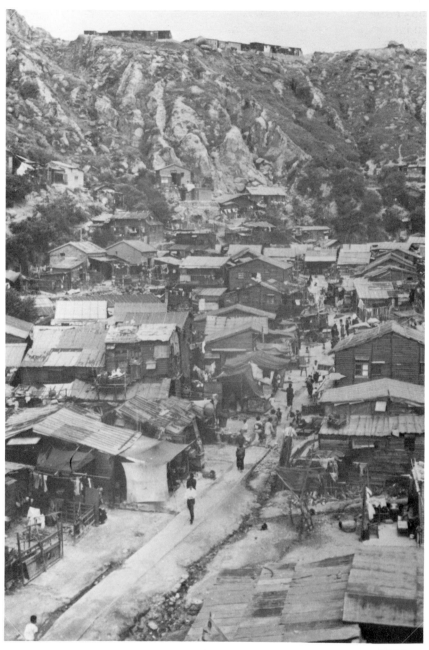

WHO (9717)

A typical shanty town on the fringe of a sprawling city

The urban population of the world, which was estimated as 1983 million in 1985, is likely to reach 2854 million by the year 2000 (an increase of 44%) and 4932 million by 2025 (a further increase of 73%) (7).

United Nations estimates suggest that, from 1975 to 1980, 54.3% of the total population increase in the developing regions was urban.[1] It is anticipated that, in the period 1995–2000, 71.5% of the increase will be in urban areas and only 28.5% in rural areas. Urban growth is in fact expected to increase as rural growth decreases to the point where, between 2000 and 2025, the rural population in developing countries will actually decrease in absolute terms (Table 2). Cumulative percentage changes anticipated in the urban and rural populations of the developing countries up to the year 2025 are shown in Fig. 1.

Urban areas in the developing regions are expected to grow over the last quarter of this century at an annual rate almost 3.7 times that expected in rural areas: an average rate of 3.48% per year versus 0.92% per year. During this period, the average annual urban growth rate will remain fairly constant (3.4–3.5%) while the rural growth rate will drop by 50% (see Table 2).

Table 2. Average annual urban and rural growth in developing and developed countries[a]

Period	Developing countries		Developed countries	
	urban (%)	rural (%)	urban (%)	rural (%)
1970–1975	3.7	1.9	1.5	−0.5
1975–1980	3.5	1.6	1.2	−0.2
1980–1985	3.4	1.4	1.0	−0.2
1985–1990	3.4	1.2	0.9	−0.1
1990–1995	3.4	1.0	0.8	−0.2
1995–2000	3.4	0.8	0.8	−0.1
2000–2005	3.2	0.5	0.7	−0.2
2005–2010	3.1	0.2	0.6	−0.2
2010–2015	2.8	0.0	0.5	−0.2
2015–2020	2.6	−0.2	0.5	−0.2
2020–2025	2.3	−0.4	0.4	−0.2

[a] Source: United Nations (7).

---

[1] Developing regions include all countries and other territories in Africa, Asia (excluding Japan), South and Central America and Mexico, and Oceania (excluding Australia and New Zealand).

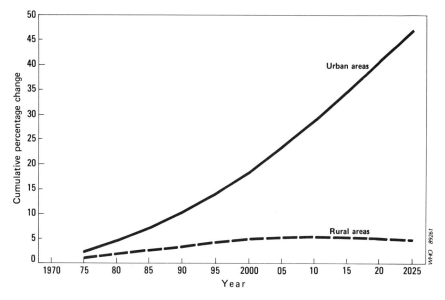

Fig. 1. Percentage change in the populations of urban and rural areas in developing countries up to the year 2025 (base: 1970)

In the developed regions,[1] the proportion of the population living in urban areas was as high as 71% in 1985. The level is projected to increase to 74% by the year 2000, and to 77% by 2025. In the developing regions, the rapid urbanization experienced prior to the 1980s is expected to continue (Fig. 2 and Table 3).

The level of urbanization, i.e., the proportion of the population living in urban areas, in the developing regions is expected to increase from 31% in 1985 to 39% by the end of the century, and to 56% by 2025.

Most major areas of the world are likely to show some increase in urban population in the future; in Africa and South Asia increases as high as 30–60% are expected in each decade from 1990 to 2020.

The publication, *The prospect of world urbanization* (United Nations), shows that the growth in the world urban population over a ten-year period (1975–1985) was 419 million. This growth was 79.4% in developing regions compared with only 20.6% in developed regions (7).

---

[1] Developed regions include countries of North America and Europe, Australia, Japan, New Zealand, and the Union of Soviet Socialist Republics.

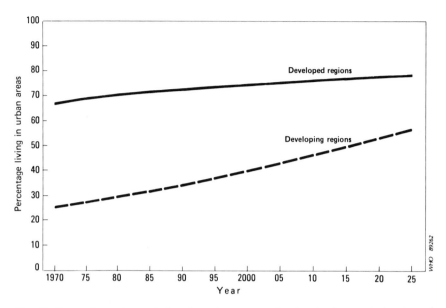

Fig. 2. Proportion of population in urban areas in developing and developed regions, 1970–2025

It is not only the size of the increase that is alarming but the rate at which it is occurring. In 1950, there were seven urban agglomerations with populations approaching five million or more; by 1970, there were 20 (Fig. 3) and, by the end of this century, there will be 60, all but a quarter of them in the developing regions of the world. By the year 2000, there are likely to be 23 cities with over 10 million people, 17 of them in the developing regions (Fig. 4). By then, Mexico City may have 26 million inhabitants, São Paulo 24 million, Calcutta 16 million, and Shanghai 14 million.

Such rapid growth is not confined to capital cities and large metropolitan areas, but also affects secondary and tertiary cities, often outstripping the ability of urban services to keep pace and forcing large sections of their populations to live in poverty and squalor. The proportion of the population expected to be living in urban areas throughout the world in the year 2000 is shown in Fig. 5.

While the developing world is undergoing urbanization at an unprecedented rate, there are major differences among countries, areas, and regions (see Fig. 6). Those with low absolute levels of urbanization, such as sub-Saharan Africa and parts of Asia, are currently experiencing high levels of migration from rural to urban areas and thus a rapid rate of urban growth. It is not simply the absolute level of urbanization that has negative consequences, but

Table 3. Estimated and projected proportion of population living in urban areas, by region or area, 1970–2025 (%)[a]

Region or area	1970	1975	1980	1985	1990	1995	2000	2005	2010	2015	2020	2025
World total	37.1	38.4	39.6	41.0	42.6	44.5	46.6	49.1	51.8	54.6	57.4	60.1
Developed regions	66.6	68.8	70.2	71.5	72.5	73.5	74.4	75.3	76.0	76.7	77.2	77.8
Developing regions	25.4	27.2	29.2	31.2	33.6	36.3	39.3	42.6	46.2	49.7	53.1	56.5
Africa	22.5	24.5	27.0	29.7	32.6	35.7	39.0	42.3	45.6	48.9	52.2	55.3
Eastern Africa	10.3	12.3	15.1	18.1	21.5	24.9	28.4	32.0	35.6	39.1	42.6	45.9
Middle Africa	24.8	28.0	31.6	35.6	39.7	43.7	47.7	51.4	55.0	58.5	61.7	64.8
Northern Africa	36.5	38.1	39.9	42.1	44.6	47.4	50.6	53.8	57.0	60.1	63.0	65.8
Southern Africa	44.1	46.8	49.6	52.5	55.3	58.2	60.9	63.6	66.1	68.6	71.0	73.3
Western Africa	17.6	19.8	22.2	24.9	27.9	31.2	34.9	38.6	42.5	46.3	50.0	53.7
Americas	64.7	66.8	68.9	71.0	72.9	74.6	76.1	77.5	78.7	79.9	81.0	82.1
Latin America	57.4	61.5	65.4	69.0	72.1	74.7	76.8	78.6	80.2	81.6	83.0	84.2
Caribbean	45.8	49.6	53.2	56.5	59.6	62.4	64.8	66.9	68.9	70.8	72.6	74.3
Central America	53.9	57.2	60.4	63.3	65.9	68.4	70.6	72.6	74.6	76.5	78.3	79.9
Temperate South America	77.9	80.2	82.3	84.3	86.0	87.4	88.6	89.7	90.5	91.3	92.0	92.6
Tropical South America	56.1	61.1	66.0	70.4	74.0	77.0	79.4	81.3	82.7	84.1	85.3	86.4
Northern America	73.8	73.8	73.9	74.1	74.3	74.6	74.9	75.3	75.7	76.2	76.7	77.3

Asia	23.9	25.3	26.6	28.1	29.9	32.2	35.0	38.3	41.9	45.6	49.3	52.9
East Asia	26.9	27.6	28.1	28.6	29.5	30.9	32.9	35.5	38.9	42.4	45.8	49.3
China	20.1	20.2	20.4	20.6	21.4	22.9	25.1	28.0	31.8	35.7	39.7	43.7
Japan	71.2	75.7	76.2	76.5	76.9	77.3	77.8	78.3	78.8	79.4	80.0	80.6
Other East Asia	47.4	53.5	60.5	66.8	71.4	75.3	77.9	80.3	82.0	83.5	84.6	85.7
South Asia	21.3	23.3	25.4	27.7	30.2	33.2	36.5	40.1	44.0	47.7	51.4	55.0
Southeastern Asia	20.2	22.0	24.0	26.3	29.0	32.1	35.5	39.3	43.1	46.9	50.7	54.3
Southern Asia	19.5	21.3	23.2	25.2	27.6	30.4	33.6	37.1	40.9	44.8	48.6	52.2
Western Asia	43.2	47.9	51.6	55.0	58.2	61.2	64.0	66.8	69.3	71.7	73.9	75.9
Europe	66.7	68.8	70.2	71.6	72.8	74.0	75.1	76.1	77.1	78.0	78.8	79.5
Eastern Europe	53.5	56.8	59.4	61.5	63.5	65.2	66.7	68.1	69.3	70.3	71.1	71.9
Northern Europe	82.4	83.9	85.0	86.1	86.9	87.7	88.3	88.9	89.4	89.8	90.2	90.5
Southern Europe	56.2	58.4	60.5	62.5	64.4	66.3	68.1	70.0	71.7	73.4	75.0	76.5
Western Europe	76.4	78.2	78.9	79.6	80.2	80.8	81.2	81.7	82.1	82.5	82.9	83.2
Oceania	70.8	71.8	71.5	71.1	71.0	71.0	71.4	71.9	72.8	73.8	75.1	76.3
Australia/New Zealand	84.4	85.3	85.2	85.2	85.3	85.4	85.8	86.2	86.9	87.5	88.4	89.2
Melanesia	15.1	17.5	18.8	20.2	21.9	23.8	26.1	28.9	32.0	35.4	38.8	42.4
Micronesia/Polynesia	32.3	35.9	38.7	41.6	44.7	47.9	51.1	54.4	57.6	60.7	63.6	66.4
USSR	56.7	60.0	63.1	65.6	67.5	69.4	70.7	71.9	72.7	73.4	73.8	74.1

[a] Source: United Nations (7).

15

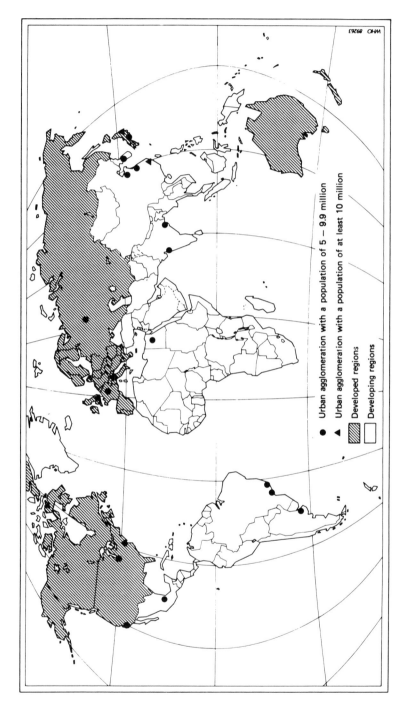

Fig. 3. Urban agglomerations with a population of 5 million or more, 1970

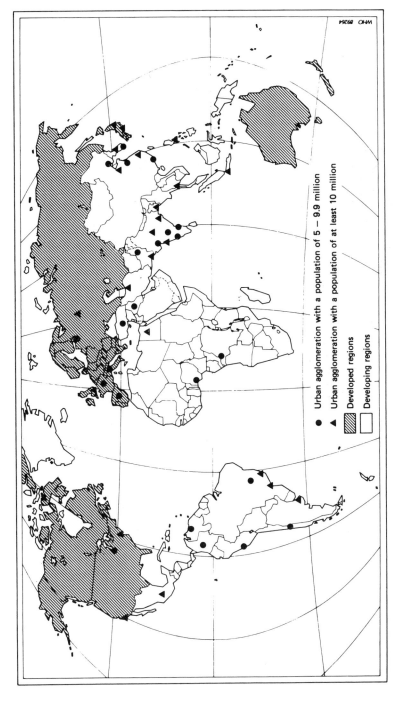

Fig. 4. Urban agglomerations likely to have a population of 5 million or more by the year 2000

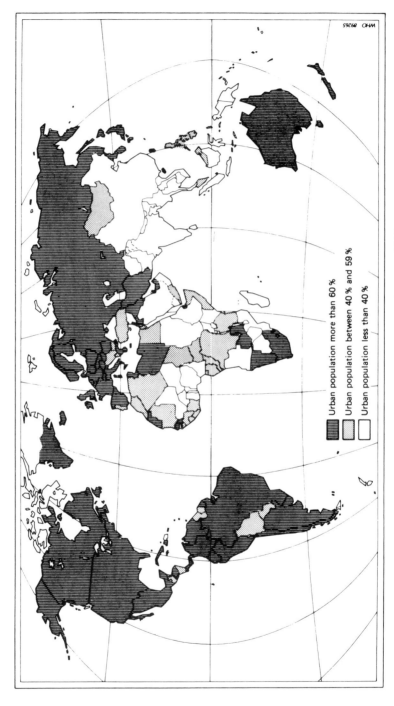

Fig. 5. Projections of proportion of population living in urban areas by the year 2000

Urban population more than 60 %

Urban population between 40 % and 59 %

Urban population less than 40 %

WHO 89265

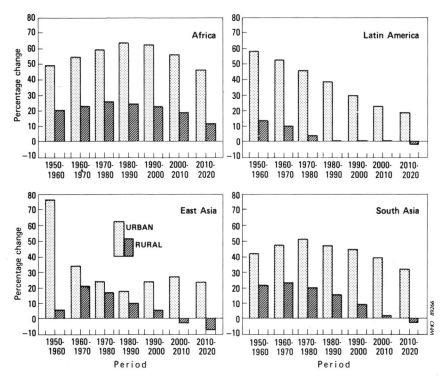

Fig. 6. Percentage changes in urban and rural population, by major areas of the world, 1950–2020

Source: United Nations (7)

also the speed with which it is increasing which causes the demand for facilities and services to grow faster than the resources available (8). Thus no developing country can afford to ignore the phenomenon of urbanization in relation to health. Those that already have high rates of urbanization may well be aware that large numbers of their urban poor lack adequate health care. Those that have low rates are likely to find that a similar problem is developing in the poorest areas of their cities at an alarming and accelerating rate.

Despite large differences in the degree of urbanization (Fig. 6), the regional trends are not so dissimilar. In every case, urban populations are growing at a far higher rate than rural populations, generally at least three times as fast. Where the urbanization level is already high, as in Latin America, virtually the whole of the region's population increase will be urban. Where it is low, as in sub-Saharan Africa and parts of Asia including China, there is expected to be a marked rise in the percentage of the total population increase taking place in urban areas. In China, for example, this percentage is forecast to rise from 56% to 113%, so that by the year 2000 the rural population will actually be decreasing in absolute terms, while the urban population will be continuing to grow at 3% per annum.

Demographic transition theory postulates that, once death rates have decreased, people will tend "naturally" to lower their fertility. Experience shows that, even if this is true, change is often very slow. In most developing countries of the Americas, for example, in spite of a decline in death rates, the situation is still one of relatively high fertility: while life expectancy at birth has increased, fertility rates have only recently begun to decline. This has the effect of increasing the proportion of the population under 15 and over 65 years of age, thus increasing the economic burden that the productive portion of the population must carry (9).

A recent United Nations report on the subject (10) points out that migration is a more important factor in urban and metropolitan growth than has been acknowledged in recent years. When the natural increase among migrants is added to net migration, it accounts for a very substantial proportion of total metropolitan growth. As about two-thirds of migrants are in the age group 15–29 years, they create a demand for employment opportunities that few cities are able to meet. However, as the report states, although migration is usually considered to impose social costs, this is not always so and, in many cases, it may benefit cities economically.

Many of the problems now being faced by the developing world have already been experienced by the industrialized countries. During the 1950s and 1960s, most of the member countries of the Organization for Economic Cooperation and Development (OECD) enjoyed a high rate of economic growth, with the urban population increasing at a far greater rate than the general population (11). In the 1970s, however, national population growth and economic growth slackened and migration flows changed. Some of the larger metropolitan areas began to lose their relative dominance and now it is the outer fringes of these cities, together with small and medium-sized cities, that have become the major foci of urban growth. The large metropolitan areas in industrial countries have also experienced a decline in population, jobs, and services, a problem that is increasingly affecting the older suburbs and some overspill towns. Thus, rapid growth in some areas is accompanied by stagnation in others. In some OECD countries, this reversal of migration has not yet occurred, and substantial migration from rural to urban areas is expected to continue.

Thus, while they vary in degree and extent, many of the difficulties of managing urban change are similar for both industrialized and developing countries. Both face common problems, which include:

— lack of effective land management;
— an insufficient supply of low-cost housing;
— unauthorized residential expansion outpacing and impeding the provision of an adequate infrastructure and public services; and
— unemployment, poverty, and all that follows in their wake.

Urbanization policies in developing countries

The usual interpretation of the process of urbanization (*12*) draws heavily from experience in industrialized countries, the key elements being the increasing complexity of technology and a shift in the demand for labour from the agricultural to the non-agricultural sector. An imbalance between demand for labour and the geographical distribution of the labour supply creates various "pushes" and "pulls" between the urban and rural areas. The primary process contributing to a redistribution of population has thus been internal migration from rural to urban areas.

The application of this model of economically induced urban growth in Third World countries is, however, questionable, because it may be occurring independently of any surge in prosperity through industrialization. Thus urban growth may not be caused primarily by the "pull" forces of economic opportunity in the cities, but by the "push" factors of rural poverty and overcrowding. Even in economically stagnant societies, therefore, there may be a significant addition to the urban population which is not absorbed into the urban economy, but remains marginally employed in unproductive fields, or unemployed. Urban growth, instead of being a sign of economic progress, as in the industrialized country model, may thus become an obstacle to economic progress: the resources needed to meet the increasing demand for facilities and public services are lost to potential productive investment elsewhere in the economy.

As reported by the United Nations (*13*), a survey carried out in 1978 indicated that only 6 of the 116 governments that responded to a questionnaire considered that the geographical distribution of their population was "acceptable"; 42 replied that it was "unacceptable to some extent"; and 68 that it was "highly unacceptable". As to the desirability of the current rates of rural–urban migration, only 3 countries expressed a desire to accelerate such migration; 23 wished to maintain it at the same level, 76 to slow it down, and 14 to reverse it. Dissatisfaction was also expressed with the continuing growth of the larger cities, the overloading of public services, the inadequacy of the social infrastructure, congestion and noise, pollution of air and drainage ditches, the scarcity of adequate housing, the abundance of slums and squatter dwellings, the inadequacy of sewerage facilities, and the lack of water, electricity, and garbage collection services in outlying suburbs.

In an attempt to cope with these problems governments have, among other measures, adopted policies to control and regulate rural–urban migration. Four approaches have been tried:

1. To improve social and economic conditions in rural areas through agrarian reforms, labour and tax policies, and so on. Considered in theory to be the most promising, this approach has in practice been only marginally successful. With a few notable exceptions (Bolivia and Costa Rica), promised land reforms have not been carried out, or only partially so (as in Egypt). The poor have rarely been provided with more land, or benefited from favourable prices for their agricultural produce. In some cases the effect has been the opposite of that intended: rural–urban migration often accelerated, as in Argentina, Colombia, Ecuador, and Peru.

2. To control migration through legislation, including residence at work-points (as in China, India, and Indonesia), slum removal, and obligatory resettlement (as in Brazil and the Philippines). The success of these measures (some of which violate Article 13 of the Universal Declaration of Human Rights)[1] generally depends on the implementation of additional measures aimed at creating adequate social and economic conditions in the settlement areas.

3. To redistribute the rural population within the rural areas (projects in Brazil, India, Indonesia, Malaysia, Nepal and Sri Lanka). Only a few of these projects have succeeded in re-locating the targeted number of persons. Inadequate infrastructure and poor communications have been among the main constraints. In addition, the projects have been costly and have covered relatively small numbers of people.

4. To accommodate migrants in urban areas through housing projects, "sites and services" schemes, and so on, as in Kenya, United Republic of Tanzania, and Venezuela (Caracas) or to

---

[1] Article 13(1) of the Universal Declaration of Human Rights states: "Everyone has the right to freedom of movement and residence within the borders of each State".

redirect them to other urban areas (satellite towns, etc.) as in Malaysia, Mexico, Peru (Lima), Republic of Korea, Senegal (Dakar), and Venezuela (Ciudad Guyana). The implementation of such projects has encountered a number of problems, and their success has differed widely. One important conclusion seems to be that, whether or not they have achieved their goals, they have stimulated more migration to the urban areas, thus aggravating the problems of urban congestion and unemployment.

Some of the projects have demonstrated that potentially effective policies can be hamstrung by bad planning, lack of coordination between ministries, poorly guided execution, and a lack of flexibility in responding to the difficulties that inevitably arise during implementation. It should also be said that for many cities the measures outlined above came too late, since the rate of natural population increase was such as to offset any of the benefits of regulation.

Nevertheless, much relevant information and experience are available in the developing countries, and they should be shared. Even unsuccessful attempts can provide a helpful starting-point, through a frank discussion of the reasons for failure. A sharing of experience is one way to improve national policies regarding rural–urban migration and to strengthen the institutions responsible for planning and implementing them. Technical cooperation between developing countries (TCDC) provides an appropriate mechanism for this purpose.

Urbanization policies and health: an example from the Sudan

The total urban population in the Sudan in about 4.5 million. No figures are available on the number of urban poor. However, the general government policy towards the low-income urban population is (a) to replan the *ad hoc* settlements around the peripheries of cities; (b) to provide a safe water supply, electricity, education, and basic sanitation; and (c) to ensure coverage by primary health care.

The main health problems of low-income urban groups are thought to be malaria, diarrhoeal diseases, respiratory tract infections, anaemia, and malnutrition, and diseases of childhood such as measles, whooping cough, and diphtheria.

All the problems of urbanization in Sudan are exacerbated by the influx of great numbers of refugees from neighbouring countries. In general little is known about the health problems of the urban refugees.

In terms of urban development, several industries have been established in urban areas, notably textile and spinning factories. These have had a positive effect in that they provide employment and regular income which improves the nutritional status of families and enables the community to participate in health-related activities. However, there is also a negative effect, namely an increase in occupational diseases, especially those of the lungs.

In Juba the low-income residents ("fourth class") comprise about 80% of the town's population of some 85 000 people. The growth rate is 9% per annum. Their most common health problems are associated with poor sanitation and water supply. More than half the town's population lacks adequate clean water, and 80% do not have access to a latrine. The Juba Area Council has embarked on a number of health projects including an oral rehydration and immunization campaign financed by UNICEF which involves the community at every stage including that of building centres. It also involves the voluntary cooperation of 23 extension workers from the Departments of Youth and Sports and Social Welfare. Drama presentations have been successfully used as an educational tool in the programme. The "training of trainers" is desperately needed, and infrastructure including buildings is still lacking. For example, immunization sessions are still conducted under trees in more than a quarter of the "councils" in Juba.

A project for the improvement of water standpipes in the town is aimed at 2000 households in the "fourth-class" areas. There are 39 standpipes, including 24 communal ones, in these areas. As well as being in poor working condition, insanitary, and unreliable, most of them lack meters. Thus a large proportion of the low-income population depends on untreated water from rivers and streams. The objectives of the project are to improve the performance, sanitary management, and maintenance of the existing standpipes.

Prepared by Dr M. A. Rahman Musbah, Director, Primary Health Care, Ministry of Health, Sudan, and Mr Christofer Gondia, Juba, Sudan, for the UNICEF/WHO Interregional Consultation on Primary Health Care in Urban Areas, Manila, Philippines, 7–11 July 1986.

The urban poor

The direct result of this urban population explosion has been a tremendous increase in the number of squatters' settlements and of the urban poor. For many countries and cities the problem is of such magnitude and urgency that the term "urban crisis" is no exaggeration (see Table 4).

In 1981, it was estimated that 79% of the population of Addis Ababa dwelt in slums and squatter settlements and, indeed, some have put the proportion even higher, at 90%. This may be an extreme case, but other major cities in the developing world are not far behind. It is not necessary to quote more figures to realize the extent and gravity of the problem. By the end of the twentieth century, the urban poor may represent a quarter of humanity.

There has been no shortage of accounts, in recent years, of the plight of those people and, while the reports have done much to create a greater general awareness of a truly dreadful situation, repeated descriptions of it are unfortunately losing the power to shock. The pattern is the same: in the underprivileged sections of the urban population, infant and child mortality rates (when they are accurately known) may be three or four times higher than the city average and there is a comparable intra-urban differential in all other aspects of health, education, and social well-being.

Few would disagree that the root cause of this urban crisis is poverty, whether it is the poverty of the rural areas that drives people to the cities, or the poverty of underemployment and unemployment that keeps them enclosed in slums and squatter settlements.

Poverty is a harsh word, but it directs attention where it is needed and there is no point in searching for a softer term. Any measure that alleviates poverty will tend to improve the health of those affected. One of the principal challenges facing health authorities, therefore, is how to participate in urban development so that the potential of all activities for improving the health of the population will be fully realized.

The term "fourth world" has been used to describe a sub-proletariat whose housing, sanitation, clothing, and food are inadequate; whose cause is not championed by politicians and unions; who have limited information, education, and voice; and who, because of indifference or intolerance, and the way that they are affected by the law and by administrative practice, are systematically prevented from exercising the rights that other people take for granted (14). From the economic point of view they are considered a burden, and from the health point of view, a danger (15). This description accurately fits the poor living in the slums and shanty

Table 4. Proportion of squatters and slum-dwellers in selected cities[a]

Region and city	Year	City population (thousands)	Slum-dwellers and squatters No. (thousands)	%
Africa				
Addis Ababa	1981	1200	948	79
Casablanca	1971	1506	1054	70
Kinshasa	1969	1288	733	60
Nairobi	1970	535	177	33
Dakar	1969	500	150	30
Latin America				
Bogotá	1969	2294	1376	60
Buenos Aires	1970	2972	1486	50
Mexico City	1966	3287	1500	46
Caracas	1974	2369	1000	42
Lima	1970	2877	1148	40
Rio de Janeiro	1970	4855	1456	30
Santiago	1964	2184	546	25
South Asia				
Calcutta	1971	8000	5328	67
Bombay	1971	6000	2475	41
Delhi	1970	3877	1400	36
Dhaka	1973	1700	300	35
Karachi	1971	3428	800	23
East Asia				
Manila	1972	4400	1540	35
Pusan	1969	1675	527	31
Seoul	1969	4600	1320	29
Jakarta	1972	4576	1190	26
Bangkok/Thonburi	1970	3041	600	20
Hong Kong	1969	3617	600	17

[a] *Sources*: United Nations, *World housing survey 1974: an overview of the state of housing, building and planning within human settlements*. New York, 1976 (document ST/ESA/30), pp. 159–164; United Nations, *the improvement of slums and uncontrolled settlements: Report of the Interregional Seminar on the Improvement of Slums and Uncontrolled Settlements*, Medellín, Colombia, 15 February- 1 March 1970. New York, 1971 (document ST/TAO/SER. C/124), pp. 21–23; *Report of the municipality of Addis Ababa to the city council*, July 1981, p. 7; International Development Research Centre, *Housing Asia's millions*, Ottawa, 1979, p. 53.

towns of most cities of the world, who are only to a small extent immigrants from other countries or members of discrete ethnic minorities; for the most part they are citizens "like the rest", of the same race, ethnic group, and religion (*16*).

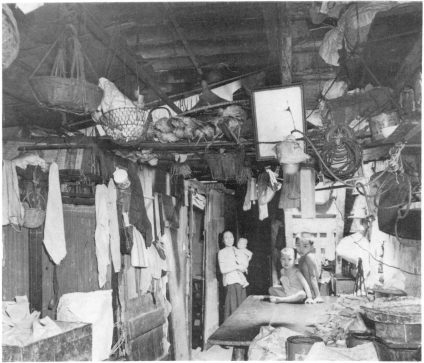

WHO (308)

Poor homes directly affect the health and well-being of the inhabitants

The measurement of poverty is difficult and may prove deceptive, especially if income is the sole criterion employed. Income statistics tend to be unreliable. A better picture can be obtained by also using non-monetary criteria, and by adding information on visible assets such as land, livestock, or houses. Although the "poverty line" may have administrative uses, it has no absolute validity: the percentage of a population above or below that line can be large or small depending on the assumptions and concepts used. The distribution of income values provides a better approach and permits the selection of a poverty line appropriate to a specific purpose. Since many policies and programmes that are intended to help the poor aim at the prevention of malnutrition, the supply of safe drinking-water, the provision of shelter and environmental services, and the provision of health care and education, deprivation should be stated in terms of these factors as well as in terms of income (*17*).

Assuming that, in the year 2000, one-half of the urban population will still be living in similar conditions, at least one billion people will be counted among the urban poor. Of these, approximately 56% will live in Asia, 24% in Latin America, and 20% in Africa (*18*). These figures, translated into human terms, forecast harsh times ahead for most of the poor living in the cities and towns of the developing world, where squatter settlements built of cardboard, wood, and flattened kerosene cans have already become a common sight and a permanent feature of the landscape.

Population movement and health: an example from Colombia

Efforts to discourage migration to the city by the rural poor of Colombia, as well as publicity campaigns to encourage a return to the land, have been undertaken to help reduce unemployment among the country's urban poor. There are also family planning projects aimed at reducing the growth of urban populations as a whole. Pressures on housing are tremendous and, in an attempt to cope with them, 40 000 units have been built in four years.

According to a national household survey carried out in 1980, 46% of all urban dwellers earn less than the minimum wage (this was US$ 90 per month in 1986). The principal health problems of the urban poor appear to be stress-induced hypertensive, cardiovascular, and cerebrovascular diseases, accidents (particularly burns), and drug abuse. There is a high homicide rate. The children of low-income families suffer mainly from enteritis, diarrhoea, and pulmonary disease. The reduction of motor-vehicle accidents, intentional injuries, homicide, and drug trafficking will require the cooperation of law enforcement agencies.

Just over half the population in Bogotá earns the minimum wage or less, with 12.4% unemployed and an illiteracy rate of about 14%. The rate of population growth in the city is 2.8%, having decreased over the previous decade. According to projections, this rate will continue to decrease during the rest of the century. However, Bogotá is still struggling under the burden created by a peak growth rate of 7% in the recent past. For example, only 52% of the city's low-income households have easy access to a safe water supply, and only 3.5% have easy access to adequate facilities for the disposal of liquid waste.

In Bogotá, for children under 5 years of age, bacterial and viral intestinal diseases and parasites, together with respiratory diseases, home accidents, and diseases preventable by immunization, constitute the major causes of mortality and morbidity. In mothers, the complications of pregnancy, delivery, perinatal illness, abortion, and cervical cancer constitute the major sources of illness and death. In 5–15-year-olds, accidents, acute respiratory illness, and eye, ear, nose, and throat ailments are the major health problems; among those between 15 and 44 years of age, accidents, and personal injuries loom largest and the homicide rate is particularly high; for those 45 years of age and older, hypertensive, cardiovascular, and cerebrovascular diseases, as well as generalized heart disease and malignant tumours, are the principal causes of morbidity and mortality.

The city has established a satisfactory statistical survey system whereby data are collected from each of the health centres and centrally correlated. Within the city health centres, the collection of information is good, but some of the marginal groups at risk outside the areas served by these centres are picked up only in surveys carried out by the medical schools, two of which place particular emphasis on epidemiology. The two principal schools involved are the Colombian School of Medicine and the Medical School of the National University.

Prepared by Dr R. A. Sanchez, Secretary of Health, Health Service of Bogotá, Colombia, for the UNICEF/WHO Interregional Consultation on Primary Health Care in Urban Areas, Manila, Philippines, 7–11 July 1986.

Health consequences of rapid urban growth

The rapid demographic growth of many cities, especially in the developing world, is stimulating the demand for resources, intensifying their utilization, and creating severe pressure on the urban infrastructure and physical environment.

The urban poor are at the interface between underdevelopment and industrialization, and their disease patterns reflect the problems of both. From the first they inherit a heavy burden of communicable disease and malnutrition, while the second brings them its typical spectrum of chronic and social diseases.

The patterns of mortality and morbidity observed among the urban poor are shaped by the socioeconomic and environmental conditions prevailing in the marginal areas to which they are confined. They are caught in a web of insecurity, low income, environmental hazards, and unsatisfied human needs. Poor health is one result, but its real dimensions are generally buried in the composite information used for overall urban–rural comparisons.

Safe water, disposal of solid wastes, acceptable housing, and adequate transport are particularly deficient in marginal urban areas. The existing service infrastructure is totally inadequate. Additional resources and development, far from providing any radical improvement, are unable to keep pace with continuing inward migration and natural population growth. Thus there is a general widening of the gap.

Environmental pollution, a widespread problem for all urban dwellers, affects the poorest members of the population most severely, since most of them live at the periphery where manufacturing, processing, and distilling plants tend to be sited and environmental protection is often weakest.

The extended family with its protective structure is often replaced by the nuclear family unit. The social structure common in the rural areas is lost in the migration process and is difficult to rebuild. This increases the vulnerability of the urban migrant. Since single-parent households, often headed by a woman, are frequent, and the need for women to work is pressing, neglect of children is almost inevitable. Even worse, many children must contribute to the family income, working under precarious conditions, in which they may well be exposed to accidents, maltreatment, and abuse.

Three main groups of health hazards simultaneously, and perhaps synergistically, operate on the poor in the cities. The first group, essentially economic in origin, includes low income, limited education, an insufficient diet, overcrowding, and insanitary conditions. The second is related to the man-made urban environment, with its industrialization, pollution, traffic, stress, and alienation. The third is the result of the social instability and insecurity that have become almost characteristic of life in certain urban areas and includes promiscuity, alcohol and drug abuse, prostitution, and child labour, leading in their turn to high rates of alcohol and drug dependence, sexually transmitted disease, and a variety of other conditions that overlap with those in the preceding group. There is also the hazard of change, especially unwanted and undesirable change, and the stress associated with it. Change often carries a physiological and psychological price-tag, for the higher the degree of change in life, the greater the risk of ensuing illness, and the more likely it is to be severe (*19*).

Specific mortality and morbidity data on infants and children of the urban poor are very limited, and most of the information

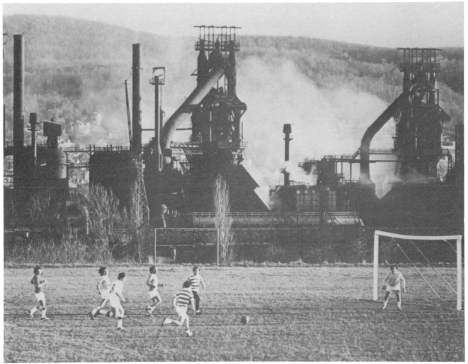

J. H. Hinman

Environmental pollution is a problem for all urban dwellers

available concerns city or country averages. However, while all members of the poor population in the cities of the developing world are vulnerable, the risks vary by age group and by sex.

Children and urban poverty

The urban environment can be particularly hostile to children. Poor housing, malnutrition, acute respiratory infections, diarrhoea and waterborne diseases, high environmental risks, lack of parental supervision and even child abandonment, early childhood labour, and other ills of urban poverty are endemic and contribute to the ill health of young children and high mortality among them. Formal education systems are often inadequate, and family and community structures in the urban environment provide little opportunity for informal education through, for example, peers and grandparents. There are limited recreational facilities. Children, particularly in single-parent families where the parent probably has to work long

31

and irregular hours for a cash income, suffer from cultural deprivation and face a conflict of value systems, which further contribute
to their psychosocial deprivation. The proportion of unattended or
abandoned children is high, and there are only limited facilities at the
community level to provide them with care and protection. Under
these conditions, children easily fall prey to the enticements and
promises of unscrupulous people. Abuse and exploitation of children
in a variety of different ways, and their involvement in prostitution
and crime, are becoming common features of the cities.

Child labour

According to the International Labour Organisation, some 55
million children under the age of 15 were working in the developing
countries in the late 1970s (*20–22*). As this estimate includes only
full-time workers and the figures are provided by the countries
concerned, it is likely to be a gross understatement. Migration of
impoverished families from rural areas to the cities is often the first
step in the process. A contributory factor is the disintegration of the
family and its abandonment by the father, which may follow from
the frustration of unfulfilled expectations. Children may be engaged
in tasks that are too strenuous for them or may have to work in
insanitary conditions. They may be forced to roam the streets, or to
live in a social environment conducive to asocial behaviour and
prostitution. Children may have to work long hours, be away from
home for most of the day and even night, be underpaid and underfed,
and receive no education or other benefits. Besides having to do
uninteresting and monotonous jobs devoid of creative and in-
tellectual stimuli, the child at this very important stage is denied the
possibility of normal mental and emotional development. The effects
on health are manifold, but not fully known and difficult to investigate, because child labour is often illegal and concealed. Malnutrition
is widespread. Exposure to toxic substances, accidents at work or on
the road, psychological disturbance, and other hazards is all too
common.

It is worth quoting a recent ILO summary of the situation (*23*):
"The ILO's research . . . has . . . found that child labour is almost
universally recognized as being undesirable, harmful for the children
themselves and to the future of their nations. Why, then, does it
persist? . . . in most cases it persists because of poverty, which
forces families to send their children out to work or compels the
children themselves to work in order to survive." The numbers of
the poor, especially the absolute poor, seem to be increasing, and in
such situations more children are forced into work and illness. The

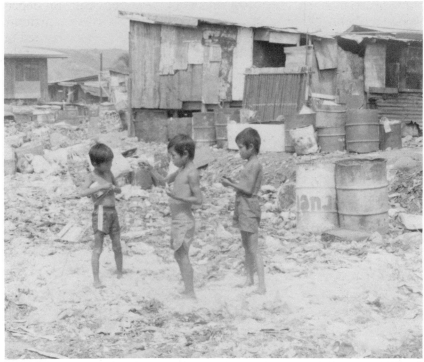

R. Maxwell

Children are particularly vulnerable to the diseases of poverty

answer to exploitative child labour and poor child health may lie in a rethinking of the causes of, and the cure for, poverty.

Street children

The numbers of street children have grown as a result of rapid urbanization, and the circumstances in which they live seriously jeopardize their health, safety, and moral welfare. They are often a product of massive migration from rural areas and the resultant breakdown of family life, or of the death of a parent, or the divorce or separation of parents. These children, now an integral part of the urban scene and estimated to be 80 million in number (24), lead hazardous lives, sometimes working at odd jobs, scavenging or begging for food, and often having to seek shelter. Some, unsupervised by adults, spend their days on the street but are able to return home at night. Others have no home to return to and sleep anywhere they can find shelter. Besides having no stable environment, they do not attend school, live hand-to-mouth (being under-

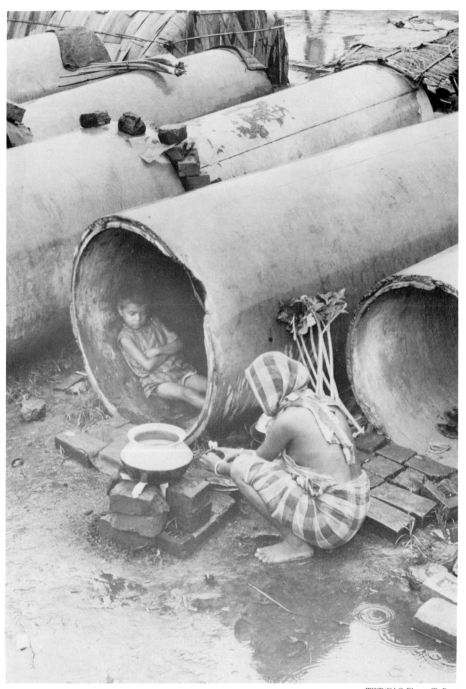

Those with no permanent home must find shelter where they can

34

nourished as a result), and are more likely than others to turn to stealing or violence as a way of living. These abandoned children inevitably suffer the consequences of lack of sanitation and clean water, occupational accidents, sexually transmitted diseases, drug abuse, crime, and all the other effects of striving to cope alone, resulting in a deep sense of insecurity and emotional conflict. There seems to be no place for them in the present social system.

Tackling the problem

In 1981–82, UNICEF sent an exploratory consultation to Brazil and, with members of the National Child Welfare Foundation, looked at what was being done for street children. UNICEF agreed to support five of the projects they saw, and the Brazilian authorities also allocated funds. Since 1982 the five projects have mushroomed into a people's movement. Social workers were picked from other communities to spend time working with the original projects and then develop projects of their own, picking up ideas here and there, as relevant. By 1984, the programme encompassed 200 communities, and today 400 communities are coordinating activities to a point at which, even if the government decided to withdraw, the movement would survive.

Two million children are under the programme's wing, and there are hopes of including all 30 million street children before the end of the century. If proof is needed of success, one need only refer to the Street Children's Congress held at the end of 1986. Four hundred children from projects throughout the country found their way to Brasilia for this event (some were sponsored by an airline company, some came by bus or boat, others hitch-hiked). They sent letters to the President of Brazil and had a meeting with members of parliament, which was covered by television and the press.

The Brazilian programme has had a remarkable domino effect. Colombia and Mexico have started their own programmes, which, if not on the same scale, are making a valuable contribution to the movement. From these countries, the idea has spread to Guatemala, Honduras, and Nicaragua. As a result of two regional conferences, one in Brazil in 1984 and the other in Bogotá in 1985, representatives from Mozambique, the Philippines, and Thailand have been inspired by the experience of the other countries to use a similar approach in their own urban areas.

Sexual exploitation of children

This is another grave problem which governments and a number of organizations are trying to bring under control (*25*). Here too, it is impossible to give precise figures, but they are high. The extraordinary growth of tourism has led to dangerous developments in this area, especially in the cities of the developing world. Thousands of girls, some as young as 12 years of age, have been sold by their parents and find themselves caught up in a network of brothels, child pornography, and drug trafficking. The prostitution of male children is also increasing. Kept in a condition of bonded labour, children of both sexes are exposed to alcohol and drug consumption and subsequent dependence, and sexually transmitted infections are widespread among them. Governments are reluctant to release information, in case it gives their countries an unfavourable image, even though they thereby make remedial action more difficult.

Child abuse

Child abuse seems to be on the increase, although some think that the figures may reflect growing awareness rather than rising incidence. Nevertheless, only a small fraction of all such abuse is reported, probably amounting to no more than 20–30% of all cases (*26*). The problem is complex and borders or overlaps those just mentioned. It includes physical abuse and excessive behaviour of different kinds (beating, burning, deprivation of food, etc.), as well as emotional deprivation, sexual, psychological, and mental cruelty, and partial or total abandonment. The slums and shanty towns of the developing countries, with all the difficulties inherent in bearing, feeding, and raising children there , constitute an environment that is all too conducive to child abuse. Tragically, there is a high concentration of abuse in institutions established for the care and well-being of young people. Child abuse may well be a self-perpetuating process, as often the "guilty" parent was abused as a child. Preventive and remedial action is hampered by difficulties in defining child abuse in legal terms and gaining agreement between law-makers and the social agencies on what is to be done.

Integrated child development service in India: Evaluation of the delivery of nutrition and health services and the effect on the nutritional status of the children

The delivery of nutrition and health services to pregnant women, lactating women, and preschool children and their impact on the nutritional status of preschool children have been evaluated in projects of the Integrated Child Development Service (ICDS) in India. A stratified random sample of 17 904 preschool children, 1210 pregnant women, and 3482 nursing mothers was drawn from 5 rural, 7 tribal, and 3 urban projects; 87–97% of those in the selected sample were available for a baseline study, and 80–98% were included in a follow-up study 20–21 months after utilization of the ICDS package of services. Considerable improvements were registered among all three categories of beneficiaries as regards the utilization of supplementary nutrition, vitamin A, iron, and folic acid, and immunization with the scheduled vaccines and toxoid. Even among children under 3 years of age there was a marked rise in coverage by all the services in the package, and a significant positive change in the nutritional status of preschool children was noted. The baseline study registered severe malnutrition (grades III and IV) in about 22% of children; this proportion was reduced to 11%, 5% and 6% in the rural, tribal and urban projects, respectively. The follow-up study showed that the proportion of children with normal or near-normal nutritional status (grade 1) had increased from 46% to 58% in the rural projects, from 46% to 58% in the tribal projects, and from 43% to 73% in the urban project area.

Adapted from: Tandon B. N. & Bhatnagar, S. *Indian journal of medical research*, **73**: 385–394 (1981).

Young people

Young people constitute a high proportion of the urban population. Some of them may have recently migrated to the city; others will have spent their childhood in marginal urban areas. Many of them, because of early employment, alienation, or lack of parental supervision, end up as school drop-outs. They are thus unable to acquire the skills necessary to compete in a limited job market. Unwanted pregnancies, illegal abortions, and sexually transmitted disease are common problems of this age group, together with malnutrition, mental disturbances, drug dependence, violence, and

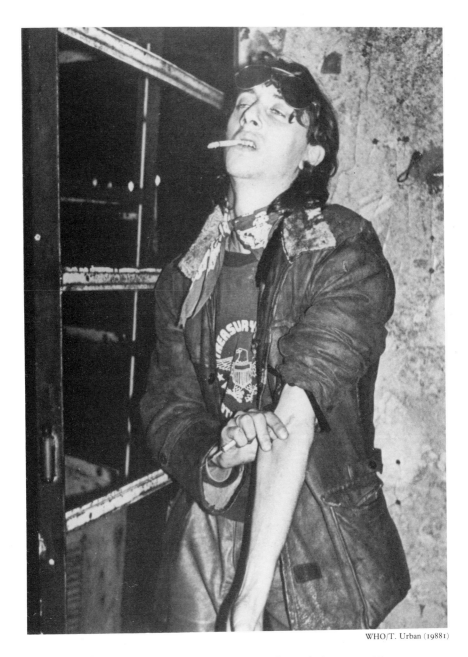

WHO/T. Urban (1988)

Drug abuse is a common problem among young people in many cities

accidents: the last two are among the principal causes of death. Faced with the inevitable stresses and strains of adolescence, the young urban poor have nowhere to turn for support. On the contrary, their circumstances, lack of qualifications, and low self-esteem combine to produce a vicious spiral from which there is often little chance of escape.

Women

A significant proportion of urban households are headed by women. Often these women have no close relations living nearby, and the nature of the marginal areas in which they live does not foster the development of other links as alternative support. A large number of women have to seek work to support their family. In the context of high unemployment, their often limited education and job skills tend to confine them to low-income occupations or to the service sector; their working hours are often long, so that their families, particularly the younger children, are deprived of care and protection. This situation also has adverse consequences for their own physical and mental health. They may run a persistent risk of pregnancy in their search for male support, they are often malnourished, and they are exposed to mental stress, sexual harassment, and abuse in searching for and maintaining a job. They tend to neglect their own health and their access to health services is limited, perhaps because such services do not exist locally or cannot be reached during their hours of opening, or because the women cannot afford the time or the cost. They tend to put their children's interests before their own.

Workers

The health of the poorer urban workers, both male and female, has always been a matter of concern. The task of making a living for themselves and their families is particularly hard in an overcrowded job market for which they are often ill prepared. Thus their main problems are the constant threat of unemployment, and the lack of opportunities and support for developing their own skills in line with the ever-changing demands of a job market that is very different from that of the rural areas. Most employment, even when available, is temporary, unskilled, poorly and insecurely paid, unprotected by legislation, and lacking in occupational health and other welfare services. At the same time, with persistently high fertility rates and the increasing number of elderly persons, these workers often have

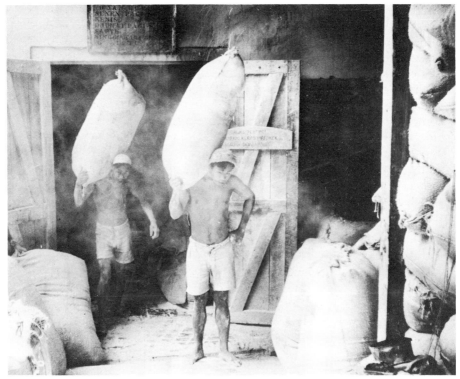

WHO (16611)

Many of the urban poor have no choice but to work in unhealthy conditions; these workers are exposed to dust which affects the respiratory tract and the eyes

many others dependent on them. Adverse health consequences have been increasingly noted in the form of accidents (reported as the leading cause of death in the age group 15–44 years in Latin American countries) among the workers themselves and generally low levels of health among their dependants. Few places provide adequate health services for lower-paid workers, and even fewer have day-care facilities for young children.

Elderly people

Demographic projections indicate that the proportion of elderly people (65 years and over) in the population will continue to increase during the next two decades. The 350 million elderly people of 1975 will become 600 million by the year 2000, and the proportion living in poor countries will rise from 50% to 70% or more. Because of intensive rural–urban migration over the last 20 years, many older people are already living in cities. Little is known of the nature and dimensions of the problems they face; however, the impact of their growing numbers is reflected in the fact that chronic and degenerative diseases are among the leading causes of death in many cities. Many elderly people live in poor socioeconomic areas and are without adequate psychosocial and economic support from family or community. Gentilini and co-workers (27) observed that whereas elderly people are tolerated in rural areas, in the city they are seen as a burden; moreover, whereas the elderly are often respected and valued in the country, they are a nuisance in the city because they lack adaptability to the "urban culture". The traditional family, which revolves around and protects the elderly, may still be found in the rural environment, but seems incompatible with urbanization.

Localization of health problems

Cities as a whole compare favourably with rural areas, in terms both of health problems and of the availability and utilization of services. However, their heterogeneous nature means that properly compiled and disaggregated information often reveals a quite different picture. It may appear from such information that the differences between the urban poor and the rural poor are not so marked, and the familiar adage of "urban better than rural" may prove to be false. Instances are becoming more and more frequent in the literature. While the lower level of reporting in the rural areas may be partly responsible for this, it seems reasonable to assume that, given a more systematic stratification of data on urban areas according to ecological and socioeconomic criteria, many other examples would emerge. A few are given below.

- In 1967, the Panamerican Study of Patterns of Urban Mortality (28), although unsuitable for an appreciation of intra-urban differentials or a stratified rural–urban comparison, already hinted at the possibility that unfavourable conditions in certain cities may result in death rates higher than those recorded in the rural areas.

- Tabulations of statistics for Thailand for the year 1970 (29) showed an infant mortality rate of 31 per 1000 live births in the Bangkok metropolitan area, while in the remainder of the country the rate was 22 per 1000. In the large slum areas of Port-au-Prince, Haiti (30), over 20% of babies die before 1 year of age and another 10% or more succumb in the second year of life; these mortality rates are almost three times those for the

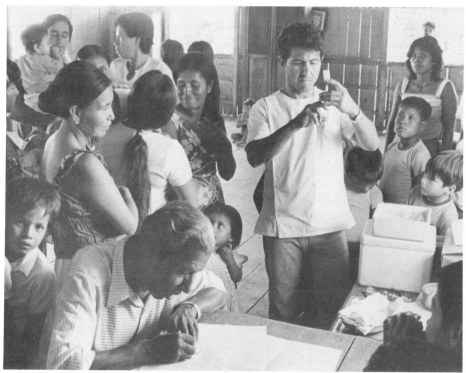

WHO/PAHO/J. Vizcarra (20259)

A tightly knit network of community health volunteers can help to ensure good coverage for immunization programmes

urban areas (while the rates for the well-to-do in the same city are comparable to those recorded in the urban areas of the United States of America).

- In Côte d'Ivoire (*31*), it was found that the average annual incidence of tuberculosis infection was 1.5%, and that this covered incidences ranging from 0.5% in the rural areas to 2.5% in the capital, Abidjan, where the rates could reach as much as 3% in the more deprived areas such as Vridi and Koumani and where the disease could strike much earlier than it did elsewhere.

- In Dakar, Senegal (*32*), one-third of the people in a periurban sample were positive for *Ascaris* infestation, while only 3 cases were found in a sample of 262 people in the rural area.

42

- In Abidjan, Côte d'Ivoire (*33*), where food supplies are considered satisfactory, there are striking inequalities between socioeconomic groups and geographical areas, resulting in lower access to food among certain urban groups than among people in rural areas. In the lower occupational strata of San José, Costa Rica (*34*), San Salvador, El Salvador (*35*) and Guatemala City (*36*) the prevalence of second- and third-degree protein-calorie malnutrition was similar to or even slightly above that found in rural groups. In Hyderabad, India (*37*), the proportion of children aged 1–7 years who presented various nutritional deficiencies was higher than it was among their rural counterparts. In certain sections of Jakarta, Indonesia (*38*), infant mortality is 85–90 per 1000 live births and there is a greater incidence of calorie-deficiency malnutrition than in the rural areas. In the Egyptian national nutrition survey of 1978 (*39*), the prevalence of stunting was found to be 15.7% and 18.8% in the disadvantaged areas of Alexandria and Cairo-Giza, respectively, compared with 27% in the rural villages of Upper Egypt and only 1.1% in a group of socioeconomically advantaged children. In four slum areas of Bangkok (*29*), the prevalence of protein-calorie malnutrition was found to be high, even in children less than 6 months old: this early malnutrition was attributed to failure to breast-feed, early weaning, or inadequate artificial feeding. By contrast, almost all infants in the rural areas are adequately breast-fed and severe protein-calorie malnutrition in children less than 6 months old is rare.

Thus, in many respects, rural migrants to the cities may find themselves worse off from the point of view of health than they were in the rural areas from which they came. Urban malaria may be prevalent, the density of the squatter population may facilitate the transmission of communicable disease, migrants may acquire a higher load of intestinal parasites than they came with, and the cost of food may make chronic undernutrition inevitable. To all of these are added the health and social hazards already mentioned.

Distinctive characteristics of urban poverty

While both rural and urban areas may share such problems as unsafe water, poor sanitation, and malnutrition, the high densities of urban populations call for fundamental, innovative solutions. Industrial pollution is a particular hazard in urban areas. Health services are, of course, much more extensive in the cities, though access to them is likely to be impeded by economic and social barriers, despite their proximity.

Local government is also far more elaborate in urban than in rural areas, which is both a strength and a weakness. Bureaucratic skills are available, at least in theory, but many poor neighbourhoods receive low priority when services are already stretched, and dealing with town and city governments can be substantially more difficult for consumers than dealing with a less sophisticated rural organization.

Although most of the settlements of the urban poor are relatively permanent and stable, they nevertheless often lack traditional community organizations. These may have to take new forms before community involvement in primary health care can be effective. In addition, lack of security of land tenure is often a fundamental problem for the urban poor, underlying their other problems and making them peculiarly hard to overcome.

Most of the major causes of death and many of the most common causes of high child mortality have clear and direct links with poverty; this is reflected in poor housing and unhealthy neighbourhoods, lacking access to decent water, sanitation, and garbage collection. Health for all cannot be achieved without adequate shelter and an infrastructure of urban services.

The facts about the urban poor are hidden because figures for their health and nutritional status are often either omitted from the statistics, or presented as aggregated data, along with the figures for more prosperous neighbourhoods. For the rapidly increasing numbers of urban poor, health conditions may in some respects be even worse than they are for the rural poor, and are deteriorating. In any attempt to deal with the needs of the urban poor, better information is required, since its absence makes it difficult to know the extent of their problems, to persuade people that these problems exist, and to formulate effective responses to them.

Another common difficulty is lack of understanding of primary health care on the part of the medical profession and the hospitals, and even the active opposition of the established health system to such care—this despite the fact that professional public health workers have nearly always played a leading part in the design of primary health care projects, the objectives of which, at the most fundamental level, are shared by everyone involved in health work.

In addition, policy formulation and planning in the health sector are often weak at the city level. Where this is the case, it will sooner or later become a crucial barrier to universal coverage. Management ability at city level is a much more important requirement than is generally recognized. Moreover, low-income groups

44

will have to develop their own representative organizations to ensure that their voices are heard.

Finally, there is the formidable constraint of lack of resources to develop and sustain new programmes. Additional funds are unlikely to be available on the scale required, so that a redistribution of resources is usually necessary, to be supplemented wherever possible by the people themselves, including the poor, however unjust this may seem to be.

Comprehensive coverage

In working towards comprehensive coverage, as opposed to initiating narrow and limited sectoral pilot projects, it is vital to overcome the problems outlined above. Conceptually, there is a sequence to be followed, from definition of needs, through the stages of experimental projects, programme development, and systematic institutionalization on a comprehensive scale, the whole process of learning and implementation taking perhaps 10 to 15 years in all. Of course it may be possible—and necessary—to find ways of shortening this process, but the pattern is worth remembering. At each stage, different criteria for measuring achievement will apply. At the project stage it is effectiveness that matters: does the approach work? At the development stage it is more a question of efficiency: can particular results be achieved at a cost that is affordable? And, finally, in the institutionalization phase, it is a matter of achieving completeness and building in resilience for the long term (40).

For primary health care to succeed, whether in an urban or a rural setting, there will have to be a change in the orientation of governments from a welfare approach to a development one, that is, not providing all the services required, but helping people to do more for themselves. It is simply not feasible to deal with the enormous problems arising in the poorer parts of the world in any other way. Above all, the attack on urban poverty and its consequences demands imagination, flair, and leadership.

Chapter 2

Reorienting urban health systems

In recent years, efforts have been made to tackle the health problems of the urban poor through the introduction of primary health care, but only on a limited scale. Numerous small-scale projects have been introduced, focusing on particular aspects of primary health care, but few of them have ventured into the area of comprehensive population coverage or included adequate provision for expansion. The time has now come when these rather restricted endeavours should be expanded so as to make a real impact on the situation in every urban district.[1]

One thing has become transparently obvious: a conventional approach is out of the question, being both inappropriate and unaffordable. If there is to be any progress, there has to be a complete change in urban health policies. The view is that only a health system based on primary health care (Fig. 7) has a sufficiently broad approach to offer a chance of success, considering the variety of geographical areas (districts) to be covered and the differing socio-economic levels of city-dwellers.

> A district health system based on primary health care is a more or less self-contained segment of the national health system. It comprises first and foremost a well-defined population, living within a clearly delineated administrative and geographical area, whether urban or rural. It includes all institutions and individuals providing health care in the district, whether governmental, social security, nongovernmental, private, or

---

[1] The term district as used here denotes a clearly defined administrative area which commonly has a population of between 50 000 and 500 000, where some form of local government or administration takes over many responsibilities from central government sectors or departments and where a referral hospital exists. Different names may be used in different cities to denote such an area: block, municipality, department, neighbourhood, etc.

traditional. A district health system therefore consists of a variety of inter-related elements that contribute to health in homes, schools, workplaces, and communities. It includes self-care and all health care workers and facilities, up to and including the hospital at the first referral level and the appropriate laboratory, other diagnostic, and logistic support services. Its component elements need to be well coordinated by an officer assigned to this function in order to draw together all these elements and institutions into a fully comprehensive range of promotive, preventive, curative and rehabilitative health activities.

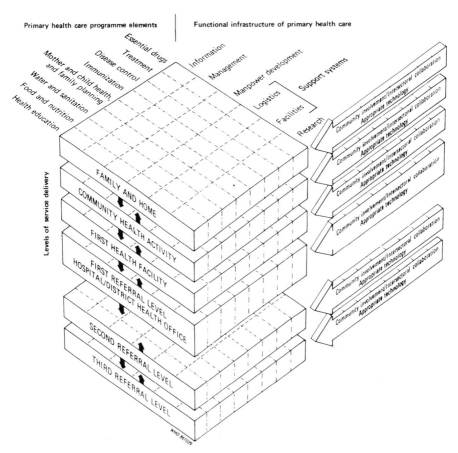

Fig. 7. Representation of the components of a district health system based on the strategic principles of community involvement, appropriate technology, and intersectoral collaboration

In this context, reorientation is crucial. Urban primary health care cannot simply be "added on" to existing services, and some fundamental changes of attitude and approach in city health systems and government agencies are needed if it is to succeed.

The primary health care approach

The primary health care approach, as defined in the 1978 Declaration of Alma-Ata, has some important strengths to offer in the urban context. These need to be widely understood:

- It helps poor and vulnerable communities to be more self-reliant in looking after their own health in the broadest sense and in determining their own priorities. Many examples could be given. China, with its highly developed urban primary health care councils, neighbourhood organizations, and Red Cross health stations provides as clear an example as any.

China: Red Cross health stations and primary health care

With an urban population of 211.87 million distributed among 325 cities, China has established a preventive urban health care system based on Red Cross health stations. In the cities, emphasis is now placed on non-infectious diseases. Hypertension in youngsters is a particular problem. The statistics from the city of Tianjin for 1984 emphasize the growing problem of chronic diseases. Some disease-specific death rates were: cancer, 86.35 per 100 000; coronary heart disease, 49.3 per 100 000; and cerebrovascular diseases, 127.71 per 100 000. Almost 23% of the population were found to be hypertensive.

Shanghai is one of three cities directly under the control of the Central Government. It has a total population of 12 million, 405 hospitals, 21 495 doctors practising western medicine, 6653 doctors practising Chinese traditional medicine, and 3190 midwives. There are 2.1 doctors per 1000 population, and the number of private practitioners is less than 600. Over 90% of the inhabitants receive medical care free of charge or at low cost.

In addition to a three-level hospital system, there are 3000 or more Red Cross health stations in neighbourhood communities. There are usually one or two health aides working in each of these stations, which were established in 1958.

Red Cross health stations deal with the prevention of disease, health education, health monitoring and the treatment of simple or minor diseases, and the health aides are allowed to prescribe certain drugs.

The stations perform tasks assigned to them by the Health Bureau, the Family Planning Committee, the Red Cross Society, the Patriotic Health Campaign Committee, and maternal and child health institutions, all of which give them some financial support. In addition, they can make money by giving certain injections and providing some medical treatment. This enables them to improve their facilities and give bonuses to their staff.

Their income is, however, mainly derived from the factories operated by the subdistricts or neighbourhoods. The Government uses some of the income from the taxes levied on these factories to support various institutions, including the health stations.

Administratively, a Red Cross health station comes under the leadership of the subdistrict administration, but it is guided professionally by the district health bureau and the subdistrict hospital.

There is a great need for more stations. Retired professional medical staff are being encouraged to work at the stations.

Shanghai is facing many problems, some of which may be similar to those in other developing countries. Generally speaking, lack of housing, inadequate transport, and pollution are the three main problems to be resolved. All have a bearing on health care.

Environmental protection and pollution control in the city have recently been improved. Two sewage treatment projects were recently completed, and diversion works from the upper reaches of the Huangpu River are under construction. This means that, in about two years, the city's drinking-water will be of better quality. Smoke pollution is being controlled by modernizing furnaces.

There is a shortage of hospitals and doctors in Shanghai. In some districts, population growth is outstripping the ability of the hospitals to cope. In all the municipal hospitals, almost 20% of the inpatients come from outside Shanghai (i.e., from other parts of South China). In specialized hospitals, this percentage reaches 60%. The everyday "floating" population in Shanghai is one million or more, so that it is very difficult for a patient to see a doctor or to be hospitalized.

The management of the hospital is another problem that needs improvement: for example, the sick-bed turnover rate is longer than in some other countries, averaging 14–20 days.

The elderly population (those over 65 years of age) has increased and in 1986 constituted 8.4% of the whole population. It is expected to increase to 11.0% in 1990, and the health care of the elderly will accordingly become a big problem. Children's mental health and nutrition are further problems to be faced.

Prepared by Dr Liu Ke-jun, Director, Foreign Affairs Division, Shanghai Municipal Health Bureau, Shanghai, China, and Dr Shan Ou-qi, Division of Urban Health Care, Department of Medical Administration, Ministry of Public Health, Beijing, China.

- It ensures that issues of a multisectoral nature are tackled, which is much less likely when conventional boundaries between agencies are adhered to. In Bangkok, for example, the primary health care approach has been expanded to encompass general development activities, which included helping residents to negotiate directly with landowners for rental arrangements that gave them legal tenure. Where the land is mainly public, as in Manila, issues of land tenure are likewise to the fore. The primary health care approach should ensure that these issues are not ignored and that ways of tackling them are negotiated.

- It can bring additional resources into the hard-pressed health care system. For example, the women's movement in Indonesia has stimulated many health-related activities in low-income urban communities.

- It can make health interventions more effective. A tightly knit network of community health volunteers can help to ensure good coverage for immunization or nutrition programmes, as was the case with immunization in Bangkok, in Visakhapatnam (India), in Manila (research and development areas), in Maputo City (Mozambique), and in several cities in Somalia. Starting from relatively low coverage, immunization rates approaching 90% have been achieved in all these instances.

Although often cited, the essential content of primary health care bears repetition, as a point of reference. It comprises at least the following components:

— education concerning prevailing health problems and the methods of preventing and controlling them;
— promotion of food supply and proper nutrition;
— an adequate supply of safe water and basic sanitation;
— maternal and child health care, including family planning;
— immunization against the major infectious diseases;
— prevention and control of locally endemic diseases;
— appropriate treatment of common diseases and injuries;
— provision of essential drugs.

By any standard, this list is long and its financial, logistic, and manpower implications are great. Primary health care is far from being a simplistic solution to the health problems of the world. However, the various components can be dealt with one at a time, in the light of local priorities, with gradual development of the health care delivery systems.

Reorienting urban health services in Indonesia

Jakarta is the largest city in Indonesia with 11.9% (769 576) of its population in the low-income category (with a food intake of less than 1700 kcal per day). The low-income population can be broken down into: temporary migrants who often return to their villages at harvest-time; slum-dwellers; domestic helps who live in relatively affluent surroundings; and nomads who do not have a permanent dwelling. The population is very hetero-geneous, with more than 130 ethnic groups.

The "five tables" system[a] has been transferred from the rural areas. Services such as family planning, maternal and child health, nutrition, immunization, and control of diarrhoeal diseases are provided in an integrated health post organized by and for the community under the auspices of the local health centre. A "Community Resilience Board" links the community with the Government and ensures intersectoral coordination, thus helping to ensure that the Government's programmes meet the community's needs. This approach has had good results especially where the generation of income has been a feature of health programmes. This has been facilitated in some areas through collaboration between the Ministry of Health and UNICEF.

[a] See Table 6, page 108

The urban primary health care programme in Jakarta also involves schoolchildren through the "little doctor" scheme, which by 1980 had trained 200 000 children throughout the country.

Most of the health officers in the city belong to the nationwide women's movement devoted to family welfare.

Surabaya, the second largest city in the country (population, 2 017 527) has similar arrangements for primary health care. There are 391 integrated health posts scattered throughout the city (about 2.3 in every *kampung* or neighbourhood).

Interesting examples of community health insurance are to be found. In one neighbourhood of 400 people, a community health scheme evolved, after the improvement of the environment by the World Bank's *Kampung* Improvement Programme. Funds were collected not only for curative health work but also for environmental services (refuse and sewage disposal, improvements to housing as regards ventilation, lighting, etc.). Ten people were selected as health officers and undertook two training sessions a week for a period of 3 months. It is notable that both the chief of this neighbourhood community and the chairperson of the local women's movement are nurses from a local hospital.

In both Jakarta and Surabaya, a multitude of nongovernmental organizations are working among the urban poor. Technology and information are generally shared between Government and nongovernmental organizations, such as the Lions Clubs, which are non-profit international associations independently managed by their local members for the benefit of the local people. Their main objective is to improve the welfare of the community, especially the lower income groups. A typical club in Surabaya has contributed US$ 39 000 to 13 health-related activities.

Critical areas for action at city level include:

— improving intersectoral collaboration "in the field";

— improving rewards and career development for health centre staff and officers;

— improving the reporting and monitoring system.

Prepared by Dr Aryanto, Jakarta Metropolitan Government; Dr Hardywinoto, Staff Provincial Health Officer, Jakarta; Dr Subakis, Jakarta; and Dr H. Suradi, Chief Provincial Health Office, Surabaya, Indonesia.

Applying the primary health care approach in the cities

In spite of the concentration of health facilities in the cities as compared with the rural areas, and the relative proximity of hospitals and other medical facilities, standards of health care fall far below reasonable minimum levels for those who live in the slums and shanty towns of the developing world. The lack of care is far graver than the overall mortality and morbidity figures for individual cities suggest, for these figures are averages, concealing the large differences between the best and the worst. Those in greatest need of medical care often have least access to it.

Municipalities cannot keep pace with the scale and tempo of urbanization and the multitude of problems that go with it. Health and other social services are not equitably distributed, nor are they planned, designed, or implemented to help those who need them most.

The primary health care strategy is based on an understanding of the roots of health problems, which often lie in the political, economic, and social realities of each nation, and attempts to find solutions that go beyond the technological treatment of problems to their fundamental causes. Thus, it also entails political decisions on matters such as employment and income, land distribution and tenure, basic education, and housing; coordinated efforts by all sectors concerned with socioeconomic development; and a better balance between "top-down" planning and the upward expression of needs, aspirations, and possible contributions by individuals and communities to their own development in each urban district. This strategy emphasizes action at the level of first contact between the people and the health system. The target is total coverage.

At the present stage, it is recognized that primary health care in the cities is faced with special problems, which include the following:

- Compared with rural areas, many urban communities lack homogeneity. In many big metropolitan cities, this heterogeneity has proved a major obstacle to urban development. More generally, individualism tends to be high in urban areas, and a sense of collective responsibility correspondingly low.

- The poorest of the poor are often the most difficult groups to reach, although their need for health care is the greatest. It is frequently the case that urban primary health care, like more conventional approaches, reaches other groups more readily than it reaches the landless, homeless, or jobless, or the street children. It would be ironic if the main beneficiaries of urban primary health care were the relatively well-off, who already have access to conventional health care systems.

- Voluntary help may be difficult to obtain in urban primary health care programmes, where households may often be headed by single parents, and may be crucially dependent on cash incomes.

- A multiplicity of agencies (governmental and nongovernmental) may well be involved in providing health care, making effective coordination that much harder to achieve.

- Resistance to fundamental changes in health care is greatest in urban settings, where medical resources are mainly concentrated. This is understandable, since nearly all human beings resist change when they do not perceive that they stand to gain by it. The opposition does not come only from professional health care workers and the hospitals. It may also come from the public and the politicians. The case for primary health care in urban settings is overwhelming, but strong advocacy is still required to explain it and gain acceptance for it.

Few countries as yet have a national strategy for urban health incorporating concepts of primary health care. Yet it is important to formulate such a strategy in order to have leverage in the competition for scarce resources, to gain a joint commitment among agencies where this is essential for implementation, and to stop inappropriate activities, that do not take priority needs into account. Several countries, such as Brazil, Colombia, Ecuador, Indonesia, Mexico, Pakistan, and Peru, have formulated or are moving towards such a national strategy, which will provide for increased investment in favour of the urban poor and promote the upgrading of slums and shanty areas instead of massive relocation.

Equity

Implicit in the primary health care approach is the goal of equity in the availability and quality of health care and health-related services. A comprehensive and searching review, at national level, of the urban situation, and an assessment of available resources, actual and potential, are essential for the development of rational and equitable policies on urban district health care. These policies should establish relative priorities, define target groups, provide for the reallocation of resources, and set health care activities in their proper relationship to other aspects of urban development. Unless

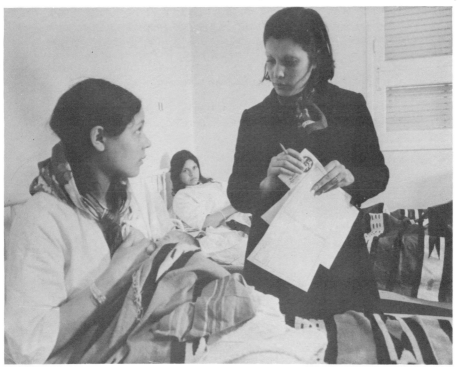

WHO/Mohr (16400)

Attention must be given to health promotion as well as curative activities: here a volunteer talks to a young mother about family planning

and until the primary health care approach makes an impact on the health system as a whole, it is likely to be seen as something for those who can afford nothing better or "a poor service for poor people".

And yet, as already pointed out, in many cities it may be the not-so-poor who have until now benefited most from primary health care. Countries with a collectivist approach, such as China and Mozambique, are notably experienced in the application of primary health care principles to whole populations. For most of the rest of the world, it is partly a matter of vigilance and of always seeking to find out whether there are disparities in the quality of services within cities and in access to them. Among the questions to be asked in any city are the following:

- Is enough attention being given to health promotion and disease prevention, including family planning, environmental planning, and behavioural factors?

- Are services accessible to all, or are there groups that are excluded or have significantly greater problems of access? Are services affordable for the poorest families and individuals?

- Is there equality in the health care available in different parts of the city or to different social or economic groups?

- Does the referral system work well in two directions: from the first contact level to the hospitals, and back to the district health systems?

- Are the content and manner of health care delivery acceptable to all?

Assessing the state of health in urban areas

How should the state of health of a town or city be measured? Certainly not just in terms of morbidity and mortality. Many other factors need to be taken into account. Thus, the extent of squatter settlements and slums, the availability of low-cost housing, the employment situation, the purchasing power of those on low wages, water supply and sanitation, communication and transport facilities, and literacy and education may be among the main determinants of health for the population.

Progress in urban development, as reflected in these factors, will lead to an overall improvement in health, even though this may not be its primary objective. Albeit indirectly, these factors are vital indicators of the health situation, and information on them is a necessary complement to conventional health statistics and data on the nature, extent, and utilization of health services.

Urban health should be assessed at a minimum of three levels: individual, community (district), and city. Of vital importance is the use of disaggregated data. As far as possible, information should be gathered and studied in such a way as to obtain an accurate picture of the situation at the district or any other level regarding economic, environmental, or social variations among the population.

Without an adequate informational framework, rational planning, effective action, and the assessment of results are greatly handicapped. The difficulty is to adjust the flow of information to the requirements of the different administrative levels concerned. Reporting often tends to go into excessive detail, with consequent delays in processing, and insufficient analysis of the data provided.

Cities are complex and heterogeneous entities, and within them health and health-related conditions vary widely by geographical area and by socioeconomic group. The information supplied to political leaders and health managers must reflect the variations, if it is to lead to a real understanding of the health problems of the population and to stimulate and guide appropriate action. Information that is not properly disaggregated may be not only meaningless but misleading, since it does not allow the true dimensions of problems and the real condition of deprived groups to stand out clearly. Thus Basta (*41*) remarks that, among the reasons why city health statistics tend to look better than rural ones, is that "squatter or slum inhabitants do not appear in the statistics (they are not 'official' residents of the city in many cases), or their inclusion is obscured by the enormous difference that exists between their status and that of the middle to high income parts of the city. Thus a very misleading average becomes the basis of that city's statistics, and averages are, unfortunately, what many look at."

In spite of the frequent abundance and variety of statistical data, the appropriate information is often not available, or else the administrators who could derive suggestions from it for significant policy changes are too busy to absorb it. While it may generally be easy for experienced city health managers to point out the "good" and "bad" areas, it is far more difficult to describe these areas and their populations, particularly the poorest, in terms of specific health hazards and conditions, effective coverage by health and other services, and community opinions and aspirations.

A systematic study of intra-urban differentials in health and health-related conditions has not been carried out anywhere in the developing world. A study of urban mortality conducted in the Americas and published in 1967 (*28*) dealt with cities in their entirety and was concerned only with intercity comparisons. Even where extensive health surveys, covering rural and urban areas, have been carried out, as in Colombia in 1970 (*42*), the study of intra-urban differentials has proved difficult because of failure to use an appropriate sample frame. Problems are compounded in what could be characterized as the standard city information system, since this generally provides an aggregation of data routinely collected for (often unclear) historical reasons, without facilities for quick retrieval and analysis. What these urban information systems should collect, process, and provide, and their relationship to the more flexible, purposeful, and probably more cost-effective *ad hoc* surveys, are matters that have generally not been delineated, though a decision on them is urgently required.

Related to the need to develop or reorient information systems for management purposes is the need to define appropriate indicators that will allow the monitoring of the various components and initiatives of primary health care delivery. The World Health

57

Organization and others have contributed to the development of material that provides a basis for selection of indicators, and several publications on the subject are available (*43–45*). Other material aims at identifying more specific sets of indicators, for example for monitoring and evaluating drinking-water and sanitation services (*46*).

The indicators selected should obviously have a clear function. In addition, they should share certain important qualities, including availability, direct utility to health workers in their daily work, low cost of collection and processing, explicit and defensible standards of definition, and, finally, discrimination in the sense that they really do differentiate important variants among the population served.

Experience shows that there are at least three distinct uses for such indicators in urban areas, namely (1) the detection of high-risk communities, (2) case and community health management by the primary health care worker, and (3) management by the primary health care supervisor. In all cases the emphasis should be on a strategy of indicator selection and data collection that will differentiate high-risk areas and groups quickly and cheaply (*47*).

The scarcity of appropriate information is specifically mentioned in reports from a large number of cities—Amman, Buenos Aires, Dhaka, Jakarta, Manila, Zerqa (Jordan), and many more—and much remains to be done before the health profiles of large, intermediate, and small cities emerge correctly. Attempts have nevertheless been made in several places to assess intra-urban differences. New methodolgical approaches have also been tried with the aim of reconciling the need for precise information with the need for speed, economy and, as far as possible, freedom from bias.

Thus, in Buenos Aires (*47*) although the information system does not permit the micro-level study of health indicators, it has proved possible to divide the city into three areas, of which the southern one has the highest concentration of health problems and the poorest levels of housing, education, and service infrastructure, particularly as regards water and sanitation.

In Ibadan, Nigeria (*48*), a survey of various health conditions, related to several socioeconomic variables in urban and rural areas, showed a gradual deterioration from "elite" urban children, through middle-class urban children, to poor urban and rural children. The poor urban children showed greater similarities to the rural children than to the other urban groups, in both health and socioeconomic variables.

Realizing its inability to locate health-disadvantaged and medically underserved persons systematically, the Manila Health Department has initiated various surveys using the neighbourhood (*barangay*) structure. Recently (1982–83), this developed into a city-wide study of the Manila health system on the basis of primary health care criteria (*47*).

Effective systems for gathering information at the neighbourhood or "patch" level have been developed in Mexico City (*49*, *50*) in a programme for its periurban population of around 5 million people. Guayaquil, Ecuador (*51*), provides an example of monitoring of child growth and symptoms by primary health care workers for the follow-up of individual cases and family action. The ability of these workers to do their jobs depends upon having quick access to the relevant information. So, in Guayaquil, the primary health care worker, who covers a maximum of 500 families, is responsible for the development of baseline information relating to these families, and the community leader will not approve payment of the worker's salary unless certain information about coverage is supplied. Experience suggests that, in addition to basic demographic data, information on the following subjects can be collected efficiently by primary health care workers with minimal training and can serve other management functions when aggregated at a higher level: certain measurable symptoms (fever, diarrhoea, etc.); the nutritional status of children under 5 years old; pregnancies and births; deaths in general, and infant mortality by cause; coverage by, and utilization of, health and social welfare programmes.

Among the urban poor, health is invariably related to income, and raising their incomes is one of the most important things to do to improve their health. Since there is no generally valid way of defining poverty within a country, let alone for comparisons between countries, it may be enough for towns and cities to use a fairly simple but consistent indicator for the purpose. For example, the number of dwellers in squatter settlements and slums, and the proportion they represent of the total population of the city may give a crude indication of the extent of urban poverty and permit comparisons between cities and the plotting of trends over a period of time.

Low-income urban districts may exist as discrete geographical entities: alternatively, low-income families may permeate some or all of the residential areas. When low-income areas can be identified as separate entities, they should be delineated using indicators that are reliable and quick to collect and that correlate well with high-risk and low-health status. In Cali (Colombia), for example (*52*, *53*), neighbourhood characteristics were correlated with infant and child mortality; this was complemented by quick, impression-gathering visits and by discussions with community leaders.

Much can also be learned from qualitative data, such as the preferences, attitudes, beliefs, and opinions of the community served and of the health workers themselves. Such information helps to illuminate and provide a context for quantitative data. It is helpful in choosing appropriate measures and identifying issues for which effective action is essential, even when these are not readily apparent from the quantitative data. Methods to obtain such data include observation, unstructured interviews, and direct discussion with interested groups. An example in which quantitative and qualitative techniques were combined comes from Cairo (*54*). In this case, it was emphasized that excessive dependence on purely quantitative information may result in an incomplete and sometimes distorted picture of the situation under study.

Thailand and the basic minimum needs approach

It is estimated that, in 1987, 25% of the Thai population were living in urban areas. In Bangkok, the low-income areas consist of (*a*) the "periurban areas" which are similar to rural areas and have a population consisting mainly of farmers, and (*b*) the "congested areas" in the inner zone. Some of these congested areas have been physically improved by the installation of walkways and drainage systems.

Poverty affects about 20% of households in urban areas outside Bangkok, whereas fewer than 10% are affected in Bangkok itself. Nevertheless, because the cost of living is lower and urban land is cheaper and more accessible outside Bangkok, a smaller proportion of the population (10–15%) lives in slums in the other urban areas of Thailand. Bangkok contains 60% of the total urban population of the country and about 70% of the slums. About one million people live in a total of 1020 slum areas. Both the total population and the slum area population were growing at the relatively slow rate of 3% per year between 1975 and 1980, less than 1% of this growth being due to migration to the city and the remainder to natural increase.

The slum areas of Bangkok have several other points of interest:

— 60% are on private land, only 4% of these being inhabited by illegal squatters;

— 40% of the slums on government land are inhabited by squatters;

— 18% of the slums, containing 35% of the slum population, have been upgraded;

— only about 25% of slum-dwellers are considered absolutely poor with income below subsistence level.

The main health problems among the low-income groups are gastroenteritis, child malnutrition, parasitic diseases, skin diseases, neuroses, and addiction to narcotic drugs.

At present, primary health care is considered to provide adequate coverage for 61% of the periurban population and 9% of the congested communities.

The health policy of the Bangkok Metropolitan Administration aims at reorienting services towards health promotion and disease prevention and extending primary health care. The main obstacles are as follows:

— Insecurity of tenure makes people reluctant to improve their dwellings and surroundings.

— The Bangkok Metropolitan Administration is legally responsible for providing health services to squatters but is prohibited from making physical improvements on privately owned land.

— Dependence on sophisticated curative services means that it is difficult for volunteers to achieve credibility.

— Economic pressures on volunteers make it difficult for them to continue as such.

— Intrasectoral and intersectoral coordination is difficult with more than 80 governmental and nongovernmental agencies involved in community development.

— It is difficult for staff to change their attitudes.

After the implementation of primary health care for one and a half years, it was evident that by itself it was not sufficient for community development. A "basic minimum needs" approach (see Annex 1) was therefore adopted, in which the processes of planning, decision-making, and implementation are carried out jointly by the community and the Government. Problems that are beyond the ability of the community to cope with are solved by the district authority, the Bangkok Metropolitan Association, or the national Government. There is a need for surveys of groups at special risk.

Prepared by Dr Sakuntanaga Pralom, Director-General, Health Department, Bangkok Metropolitan Administration, and Dr Vutipongse Prakroom, Director, Primary Health Care, Ministry of Health, Bangkok, Thailand.

In some countries, a number of indicators of social development have been introduced. The choice varies from city to city. Bangkok currently uses 33 and Manila 6 indicators to monitor the quality of life. Sometimes (as in Bangkok) the indicators include attitudes and other subjective factors, as well as objective ones like mortality and morbidity rates. The Bangkok strategy, which relates its choice of social development indicators to basic minimum needs and sets future targets, is documented in Annex 1.

In the main, maternal and child health programmes appear to provide the most reliable data. Infant mortality is for the moment the single most commonly used indicator in assessing the relative health status of different communities and in monitoring progress.

Data-recording needs to be firmly anchored in the home. The basic record for the whole family should, whenever possible, be retained by the family, which can then show it at any health facility whenever a family member is sick, even if the family moves. A good example is provided by the Manila project in which child growth is recorded by the mothers, who keep the basic record and are aware of the significance of the data. In Manila also, basic health data are carefully collected by community health workers and aggregated at the health centre level. Such a system needs careful supervision if its accuracy is to be maintained in the long term.

The data also need to be well used at the district level, as well as centrally. This is relatively rare, even where data collection is good. Yet quite a simple analysis, visual presentation, and discussion of the data can provide invaluable information about the relative priority of each community's health needs, on which decisions can be based. Simple analysis of the basic data can help track different needs in different neighbourhoods and assess progress over time. If primary health care is the right approach, the benefits should show up unambiguously as measurable improvements in health status. The community and the politicians have a right to information that will enable them to see whether such improvements may legitimately be claimed.

Community diagnosis (through, for example, people's own assessment of relative poverty and of priorities) can provide a cheap and valuable complement to data on activities. Surveys have an important place also, because they can help jolt everyone out of the assumption that activities are maintaining their relevance to needs.

All too often, information within the same city, or even within the same neighbourhood or district, is in different formats and available from different agencies. By contrast, Colombia has a good system for central data collection, although the data are still not regular or uniform. In most cities, methods for information referral and analysis need to be reviewed, systematized, and standardized. Computers can help, as in the standardized reporting systems of Colombia, Manila, and Somalia.

Finally, information systems for primary health care in urban districts should be judged by their ability to disaggregate residential neighbourhoods according to the health status of their inhabitants, their social needs, and the extent to which these needs are satisfied, and thus to guide managers in allocating or reallocating scarce resources equitably. Political will, managerial pragmatism, and information for action are all closely related. As Rosenblatt reminds us (55), "Archimedes said he could move the world as long as he had a long enough lever: he pointed out, too, that he needed ground to stand on." In the case of the urban poor, the lever may be political will; the solid ground is reliable, discriminating information.

Health systems research

Information is essential for adequate understanding and appropriate management. Pragmatic health systems research contributes to the generation of appropriate information, especially when such information cannot be derived from the routine statistics. It is concerned with the identification of health problems, their determinants, and their priority, and the formulation, testing, monitoring, and evaluation of innovatory measures. Research on disease prevention should be given priority, because only preventive action makes it possible to attack prevalence by reducing incidence (56). Health systems research is culture-linked and hence, although the same methods can be widely used, the results are often not transferable. It should therefore be included in the activities of all urban health systems and not confined to specialized groups in a few centres.

Because of the political, social, and economic implications of its results and the threats it may pose to vested interests, health systems research is often a sensitive activity and health administrators may be reluctant to authorize it. Alternatively, they may not recognize the need or have the resources for it. Here, as pointed out in 1984 by the Thirty-seventh World Health Assembly, the initiative or collaboration of the universities is crucial, in view of the multidisciplinary nature of such research. A discussion of, and suggestions for, health systems research can be found in recent WHO publications (57, 58). There is a need to investigate issues such as the following:

— the consistency of urban health policies, plans, and programmes with the principles of the primary health care strategy;

63

— intra-urban differentials in health and health services, their determinants, and their implications for the urban district health system;

— the coverage of the poorest areas and population groups by health and other relevant services, and the efficiency and equity of the referral system and of the current structure;

— alternative models of neighbourhood health development programmes and identification of constraints to their correct functioning and expansion;

— inhibiting and facilitating aspects of urban health legislation;

— characteristics, problems, effectiveness, and potential of the urban community health workers (or health promoters);

— availability of emergency services in marginal urban areas;

— the social adaptation of migrants to the city, and the health implications of their adaptation or failure to adapt.

An urban strategy in Guatemala

The population of Guatemala is 7 926 692 of whom 3 180 000 (40%) constitute the urban population; mothers and children form 65% of the total population. The growth rate is 2.7%, the birth rate 37.1 per 1000 inhabitants, and the fertility rate 166.8 per 1000 women between 15 and 44 years of age. These figures are characteristic of a young and rapidly growing population.

The health indicators of the country show a general mortality rate of 9.6 per 1000, a maternal mortality rate of 11.2 per 10 000 live births, and an infant mortality rate of 64.9 per 1000 live births.

A large proportion of the urban population lives in Guatemala city, and this proportion is increasing rapidly.

Within urban areas it is possible to distinguish several population groups, with widely varying rates of infant mortality ranging from 33 per 1000 to 113 per 1000 among the children of illiterate women in the lowest socioeconomic group. The risk of child death is greater among the inhabitants of marginal areas on the outskirts of the city and in the centre; such areas contain 20% of the total population, or 240 000 inhabitants. The chief morbidity problems reported among children under 5 years of age in the marginal urban areas are acute respiratory infections, gastrointestinal complaints, diseases preventable by immunization, perinatal diseases, and malnutrition. Low birth-weights were recorded for 16.6% and 15.8%, respectively, of babies born in the maternity wards of two hospitals serving the marginal areas.

The available indicators show that the living conditions of the "marginal" group are clearly inferior to those of the rest of the urban population; 87.9% of them are illiterate, and they have an unemployment rate of 62.4%, while the 37.6% who do work are underemployed.

Despite this situation, there is a definite political will to tackle many of these negative factors. Thus it was recently planned to augment the support of the Government and the international collaborating agencies for projects aimed at:

— expanding maternal and child health care in the marginal areas; and

— integrating the various components of primary health care in urban areas.

To achieve this a concentrated effort, based on the following strategies, is required:

— a primary health care approach, laying stress on maternal and child health;

— active community participation;

— concentration on child survival;

— concentration on activities that can be quickly implemented;

— emphasis on low-cost and high-impact measures;

— a multisectoral and multi-agency approach;

— integral care as part of teaching activities;

On the basis of these strategies it is proposed to concentrate efforts on six main areas:

— follow-up of child growth and development;

— oral rehydration therapy;

— breast-feeding and infant nutrition;

— immunization;

— implementation of a risk approach to maternal and child health;

— prevention and control of acute respiratory diseases.

Prepared by Dr Hilda de Molinaheal, Department of Health Services, Guatemala.

Priorities in introducing primary health care

The introduction of primary health care in a rural area requires a tremendous effort and resources for assessment, programme development and delivery, logistics and referral support, and monitoring and evaluation. In the towns and cities, with their large squatter and slum populations, the difficulties should be less severe, if the resistance to fundamental change mentioned earlier can be overcome, because more trained personnel are available in the cities and communications are much easier.

Priorities should be set on the basis of (a) the most important causes of mortality and morbidity in the short run; and (b) achievement of total coverage. When these criteria are applied, the resulting priorities will depend on the prevailing epidemiological and socio-economic conditions. However, the following measures are almost universally required: encouragement of breast-feeding and appropriate weaning practices; diarrhoeal disease control, including oral rehydration; basic immunization of women and children; control of acute respiratory infections; monitoring of child growth, health, and development; community health education with special emphasis on the education of mothers; and supplementary feeding in the context of acute food shortages.

In the short run, emphasis on these measures will rapidly reduce infant and child mortality and morbidity. This initial success should in turn trigger off the development of more complete health care delivery systems at the primary, secondary, and tertiary levels.

Wider deployment of pragmatically trained community health workers is an important—and often essential—step, as is their integration with more highly trained and specialized professionals in community-oriented, multidisciplinary health teams with strong support and referral networks.

The strengthening of municipal health departments or equivalent bodies in each urban district, together with a broadening of their outlooks and skills to fulfil the requirements of the primary health care strategy, is a necessary supporting step. So, too, is the improvement of management at all levels.

There also needs to be a recognition of the fundamental role that hospitals, most of which are located in the cities, can play in support of primary health care. Both within and outside the hospital, increased awareness of this role should lead in turn to better and more community-oriented hospital services, medical schools, and nursing schools.

Another requirement is a broader approach to health promotion and disease prevention that will extend responsibility for health to all

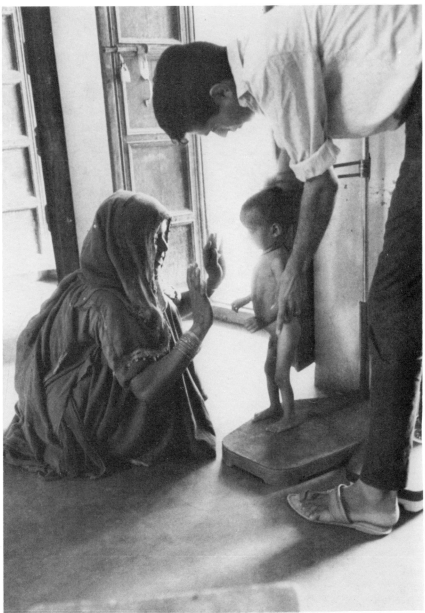

WHO/Claude Huber (12879)

Regular monitoring of child growth and development is an essential component of primary health care

sectors, agencies, and individuals in the city and emphasize multisectoral action at the district and local levels, giving priority to the urban poor. Mechanisms are needed to ensure coordination between the relevant departments, including those dealing with education, public works, industry, commerce, housing, transport, and communications.

It is vital to promote community organizations that will assist immigrants when they arrive in the city and when they move from one urban district to another or even within a district, assess community needs and make them known to government and other organizations, initiate projects to alleviate particular problems of specific population groups, secure external resources, and mobilize local action and self-help.

Obviously not everything can be done at once. It is, therefore, tempting to think that there must be some generally applicable guidance, based on experience, about the sequence of activities to follow. "Concentrate on water supply first, and sanitation second" is the type of advice that some administrators might wish to have. But that is a simplistic and unnecessarily limiting approach. The general view among people with substantial experience of primary health care (59) is that it is by no means such a simple matter. Different environments warrant different priorities. Different communities may well make different choices. While there is, in any case, an important sense in which it does not matter much where one starts, since urban primary health care comprises a cycle of interdependent activities, it makes a great deal of difference to start with the people's priorities.

Three principal points emerge:

1. The main activities are interdependent, and any worthwhile activity can therefore be taken as a starting-point.

2. Informed community choice is what matters, and therefore priorities are best stated in terms of *processes*, for example:

   • organize initial training for community health workers, the community, and the relevant professionals, including development workers;

   • establish good and simple information systems so that people can make informed choices;

   • arrange a structured debate about choices, involving the community, the professionals, and relevant government officials;

68

- let the community decide, with technical advice, its priorities and broad strategy, and what it wants to do first;

- build up logistic support.

3. In the end, primary health care is bound (sooner rather than later) to be a comprehensive package of services in urban districts including, in whatever sequence or priority, water supply, sanitation, shelter, nutrition, basic health care, employment, and education.

Resources: money, people, and imagination

Urban areas already have a large share of the available national resources for social care, including health. It is therefore unrealistic to expect great increases in resources for health. The challenge for governments and other authorities is to devise ways of using the available resources more equitably and effectively, and to mobilize appropriate community action and support from other sectors.

As the national health budget is often largely absorbed by the maintenance of existing institutions, programmes, and services, the room for manoeuvre is usually small. But, with encouragement and a little imagination, most medical and health workers, even those in specialized fields, can find a way of contributing, directly or indirectly, to an improvement in the state of public health. For example, in Malawi, the review of the health system structure and analysis carried out for the national health plan (1986–1995) showed that potential savings in costs in the largest hospital amounted to approximately 35% of its total annual operating budget, i.e., about 7% of the net total operating budget of the Ministry of Health. In the light of this, the possibility of substantial savings from increases in efficiency elsewhere in the Malawi health system is being examined.

The call for a reallocation of resources and a shift towards primary health care is, therefore, an appeal as much for a change in attitude as for increased funding.

If the health problems of some urban districts seem almost overwhelming, the potential resources are also considerable, though often unexploited or underused. If primary health care cannot be introduced where there is a defined high-density urban population, it must seriously be questioned whether it can succeed anywhere.

On the basis of current experience, as presented at a UNICEF/WHO Consultation in Manila (59), the following simple and straightforward advice may be given:

- Mobilize *all* available resources, including the various levels and departments of government, the private sector, nongovernmental organizations and international agencies, and the public. It is surprising what any one element in this combination can produce: for example, in Baroda (India), a nongovernmental organization mustered US$ 30 000 for urban primary health care within a few days, through an umbrella fund-raising organization. Any proponent or manager of urban primary health care programmes has to be an entrepreneur.

- Consider what it is fair to require from the health care professions as a contribution to primary health care in poor rural or urban areas. In Indonesia, for example, newly qualified doctors are required to work for two years in the outer islands on government service (5 years in Java) and the Philippines has a voluntary scheme of 6–12 months' public service.

- Do not ignore the resources of the community itself, however poor it is. By no means all deprived communities are poor in cash terms. In Manila, health insurance to pay for medicines is linked to credit unions for small loans. In Thailand, the purchase of health cards is a kind of prepaid insurance securing faster and better service for card-holders. And, in Hong Kong, health maintenance programmes are based on participation and contributions from the local community. Communities that are without cash can often provide equally important resources in the form of time, skills, and sheer pertinacity. Moreover, an important aspect of community development and self-respect is that people do what they can for themselves. Income-generating schemes (of which there are some modest examples in Manila) are an important adjunct to primary health care in poor communities.

- Persuade politicians, governments, public agencies, the medical profession, and the hospitals to reallocate the relatively modest resources required to make primary health care programmes feasible. While the basis of the financial calculations varies between projects and programmes, the available evidence suggests that, in many parts of the world, $1–5 per head will pay for most components of primary health care in both urban and rural districts. One suggestion is that in countries where money is allocated to cities on a programme basis, central and provincial governments could make statutory provision for cities to spend at least a defined proportion of their budgets on primary health care programmes.

70

● A strong information, education, and communication strategy may help tilt the political will towards primary health care. The attitudes and orientation of senior politicians and government officials at the policy-making level can be changed by bringing effective primary health care efforts to their notice. For example, Colombo's programme to convert bucket privies into latrines (within three years, 3800 out of 5200 privies were dealt with) was triggered off by letting politicians and administrators see how a similar programme was carried out at Patna in India.

Orientation, education, and training

Training needs go far beyond the formation of new categories of personnel, such as neighbourhood health workers or health promoters. For the foreseeable future for more than half the population of the world, the solution of the most pressing health problems and the delivery of essential services will depend largely upon the skills and efficiency of "a myriad of personnel who make the policy and carry out the tasks that keep cities and towns working"(60). Needs include the orientation of political leaders, the training of managers at various levels and of people who work in the community, and the continuing education of various other categories of personnel. New training programmes have to be developed for community health workers, traditional birth attendants, and others, and established training programmes (in medical and nursing schools, etc.) restructured. Yet what is being done is a minute proportion of what should be done. Without even considering the much greater needs that lie ahead, the process of seriously identifying training needs, estimating the necessary resources, assessing what already exists, formulating training activities and developing the necessary instruments to carry them out has hardly started in most places. Because of the specificity of health problems to local conditions, training must be related as closely as possible to needs; local resources must be mobilized; universities and other training institutions must be involved; and links must be established with related training programmes established by other sectors (60).

In the reorientation of health workers for primary health care, it is essential to take a broad view encompassing the major factors and forces that influence and determine behaviour. Continuing education cannot be considered in isolation. The reorientation of health workers is bound to fail if it is considered merely as a series of refresher courses, without any attempt being made to restructure their basic education (in terms of curriculum content and educational approaches) and to adjust managerial functions and organizational procedures.

Since the present fragmented approach leaves too many issues relating to manpower training and management unresolved, an integrated national policy on training for primary health care is called for. Such a policy becomes essential when critical issues are not resolved, when solutions are known but not applied, when implementation is uneven and unsatisfactory, when lines of responsibility are unclear, and when some of the main groups concerned are failing to support primary health care.

The formulation of an integrated national policy in this area would normally lie with the training division of the ministry of health, but a training institution could also be charged with the task. Politicians, legislators, educators and trainers, high-level administrators, professional bodies, and nongovernmental organizations all have to be involved, and it will take considerable sensitivity and persuasive powers to get them to collaborate in setting goals and to work together with a clear sense of direction.

A clear statement of issues and alternatives is needed, as well as an evaluation scheme for determining how policy is translated into implementation at different levels.

The following major factors should be included in the reorientation of health workers: advocacy, information flow, intersectoral linkages, applied health systems research, information support, and the management of networks.

An example of a university hospital and improving urban health

The Aga Khan University in Karachi, which is the first private university in Pakistan, is making a serious attempt to approach the concept of a health-for-all university. Improvement of the health of people of Pakistan is the university's main objective. To meet this objective, the Department of Community Health Sciences is training young doctors and nurses for leadership in dealing with the health and development problems of Pakistan, particularly in the deprived population, and developing field programmes that are effective in addressing the most intractable problems of urban and rural populations through the organization of health systems based on primary health care.

In this respect, 20% of total curriculum time is allocated to the study of community health sciences which is strongly community-based and problem-oriented.

To avoid teaching primary health care as mere theory, there is a need for living examples of primary health care modules that are close to the principles of health for all—universal coverage and care according to need, community involvement, an information system for monitoring and evaluation, some cross-sectoral activity and affordability in terms of local resources. Five such modules have been developed in urban settings covering a population of 50 000.

There is also collaboration between the University and the local government to improve health services at the district level.

In the north of the country a joint effort with the Aga Khan Health Services for Pakistan is under way to develop a primary health care system for the entire population.

The primary health care module is a three-tier system:

— Community health workers are the first-contact health providers. They are women from the community who are motivated and willing to work for the improvement of health status. They visit assigned homes in their areas on a periodic basis and identify individuals at high risk, such as malnourished and nonimmunized children, and pregnant women. They collect information and maintain close links with the community.

— A lady health visitor supervises the community health workers and supports them in the surveillance of those at high risk, takes care of more difficult problems and collects information on prevalence of malnutrition, number of births and deaths, etc.

— Community health nurses were recently introduced in Pakistan. Together with the community health doctor, the nurse supervises the community health workers and lady health visitors and provides clinical and managerial back-up. The nurses analyse the community data and make interventions accordingly.

The referral system links the community with a base hospital which in turn supports primary health care. The involvement of the community is encouraged at all levels.

Though health-related issues are used as entry points, efforts are under way to expand activities to other sectors for socio-economic transformation.

Prepared by Shirin N. Mohammad, Farid Midhet, Rafat Hussain, and Asif Aslam, Aga Khan University Hospital, Karachi, Pakistan.

Since the concept of primary health care is often not properly understood, efforts must be made to explain it to a wide range of people and institutions, in particular political, religious, and community leaders, teachers, middle-level civil servants, technical officers, professional associations and nongovernmental organizations.

A series of short workshops or seminars, backed up by appropriate brochures and other easy-to-read material, can do much to create better understanding on the part of the above groups and the broader public, particularly if suitable media coverage can be arranged.

A striking feature of the responses of various people to questions about primary health care is that there appears to be a block in the flow of information at mid-level management. Technical documentation often does not reach the health workers for whom it is intended and, unless it is personally addressed to the individuals concerned, there seems to be little chance that they will receive it, as it is likely to get held up somewhere in the system. It might be preferable to prepare brief, easily understandable, and clearly written material on selected issues in primary health care, send it directly to health workers, with copies to supervisors, and secure regular feedback from the recipients regarding its appropriateness and usefulness so that their interest can be sustained.

Among the fundamental changes required by primary health care is the reorientation of the attitudes, approaches, and skills of people within the health system. In Manila, health personnel at all levels have initiated a process of reorientation and development of skills that will enable them to implement primary health care. A series of technical and managerial learning modules is now being followed by the staff. These cover: new health techniques; developmental skills to help communities organize themselves; planning and training skills that involve community participation; information analysis (so that staff can digest, present, and discuss health levels and trends); and managerial and leadership strength.

Each country has institutions and people working in relative isolation, and it is essential to establish formal and informal networks so that these resources can be mobilized and utilized fully. A national health development network should be established, encompassing service, training, and research institutions, professional bodies, and nongovernmental organizations.

A programme of study tours or visits to the various institutions should be organized to enable health workers to assimilate different kinds of experience at first hand. Regular meetings should be held to identify problems and common or complementary activities, and to develop a unified approach to the promotion of primary health care.

74

Financing primary health care in urban areas

The expansion of primary health care projects to achieve universal coverage in urban districts is going to involve substantial effort and considerable sums of money. Who will pay—the government, the municipality, the community, or all three?

A searching examination of health needs and the ways in which they may be met could lead to a reorientation of existing urban health services towards primary health care and, in theory at least, a reallocation of funds and resources for this purpose.

However, there are probably few situations in which such a drastic change would be immediately acceptable, for there is likely to be formidable opposition from those whose interests are threatened, despite the strength of the moral and economic arguments for extending essential health care to the whole population.

Thus it seems that a substantial part of the resources, financial and otherwise, required to build up primary health care systems will have to be found by the communities themselves. They will also have to help mobilize support for the necessary changes in the established patterns of allocating health care resources.

On a per capita basis, the resources required to transform the health of the urban poor are not large. A cost-benefit analysis for the Guayaquil project suggested that US$1 per head per annum could yield substantial benefits (51). But even such a modest sum, when multiplied by a large number of people, becomes formidable. Obtaining funds—and more importantly the personnel and supplies for which they pay—is therefore a matter that cannot be ignored.

The resource problem is aggravated by the heavy commitments of existing services that rarely reach the urban poor and frequently concentrate on relatively costly activities. Changing the balance so that resources are deployed intelligently, humanely, and cost-effectively could be expected to be easier in more prosperous times when a real annual increment is available for the development of new services.

Finding financial resources for pilot projects or innovative experiments does not, on the whole, present a problem. Even in these difficult economic times, a convinced supporter in a position of authority within a government can generally redirect finance on the scale required. If not, there are usually other possible sources of help, such as nongovernmental organizations, the churches, and the international organizations. A greater constraint than lack of money —particularly in gaining the confidence of a community that is deeply suspicious of authority, as is often the case—may be a shortage of people with the skill and experience needed to carry out the proposed projects.

It will probably prove even more difficult to sustain these projects on a long-term basis, as part of the established pattern of services; to move from pilot schemes towards comprehensive coverage; to change the priorities of the health care system as a whole; and to alter the ways in which people think. Here, nongovernmental and international organizations cannot fill the vacuum. Only the country and city concerned can do so, although a continuing contribution can be made by these organizations through, for example, advocacy and bargaining vis-à-vis the authorities and the professions; and through "networking", educational activities, and support for those directly involved in primary health care.

The transition from limited projects and isolated, local examples to a continuing, comprehensive, and expanding pattern of primary health care will be facilitated if people consciously prepare for it from the beginning. For example:

- A baseline survey will help to establish sound epidemiological evidence on which targets can be based and programme effectiveness demonstrated.

- The more the primary health care service is "owned" by the community concerned, the greater its chance of survival, partly because even the most deprived communities are not totally without resources for things they value highly, and partly because their own leaders will at times be able to exert political influence.

- The more modest the recurrent cost of the service, compatible with quality and effectiveness, the better. Moreover, ways are being developed to enable community health workers themselves to generate resources to sustain the service on a continuing basis. Whenever possible, primary health care initiatives should be linked to other community projects that generate employment and income.

- Projects that are designed on a modular basis can be readily extended within the same environment, as resources become available.

- It may be possible by persuasion, or by official intervention, to obtain some degree of financial support from industrial enterprises situated alongside poor residential neighbourhoods. At the very least, they should be subject to regulations to ensure that they do not make the health situation worse through environmental pollution. More prosperous residential neighbourhoods and voluntary organizations may also provide some help, for example, by sponsoring some aspect of the primary health care service.

● Injections of resources for primary health care should be related to specific short-, medium-, and long-term objectives so that value for money can be demonstrated and the intended changes of balance within the health system assessed.

Urban health departments

Effective support for primary health care is likely to require changes in urban health departments. More important than organizational restructuring is a general change in attitudes, since a fundamental shift in values, strategy, and approaches is involved. In most cases, reorganization is not an immediate requirement, but should rather be left to evolve when there is already some record of initial achievement. Various alternatives have been discussed in a recent WHO publication (61). Collaboration and communication depend fundamentally on personal qualities and personal contacts. They also depend on a sufficient concordance of aims among all those concerned.

An example is provided by the radical changes that have been taking place in the Municipal Health Department of Manila (Manila Health Department, unpublished information, 1983). Several steps are involved, including: a drastic shortening of the lines of communication between the districts and the operating staff in the field; new roles for public health nurses, who are expected to work more closely with community leaders; coordination of field services under the supervision of a team leader; strengthening of the city's district information system notably in its capacity to assess needs dynamically, monitor progress, and evaluate the effect of health measures; improved training programmes for the basic and continuing education of community health workers; and, finally, greater involvement in meeting the basic needs of the population (food, water, sanitation, housing, employment) through intersectoral action.

A reorientation of municipal health departments has been undertaken in several other cities. What seems to be needed is not a major reorganization of departments nor, still less, the creation of a "primary health care" office or programme. It is rather a change of mentality that is required and the application of primary health care concepts to all aspects of the departments' work. Such a change entails a greater social orientation of the hospital system, an improved ability to convince and to respond, and the prestige to deal with departments outside the health sector so as to mobilize resources where and when needed. It also calls for alertness in recognizing and using every possible opportunity for concerted action, an ecological–epidemiological approach to health development, and greater emphasis on prevention. Finally, there has to be a reorientation of medical and other types of health personnel that should start with their basic training.

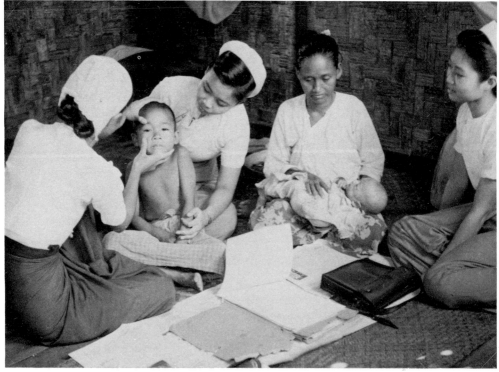

WHO (4184)

A public health nurse, accompanied by two students, uses the opportunity afforded by a postnatal visit to examine the other children in the family

Lagos, Nigeria: involving the university hospital

Health care in Nigeria currently concentrates on the rural population, which constitutes 70% of the country's estimated population of 96 million.

In Lagos, which has a 14% growth rate, 25% of the inhabitants belong to the low-income group. Officially, the low-income population comprises those earning less than about US$ 2000 per annum. The official minimum wage for the country is fixed at about US$ 125 per month.

The main health problems of the children in the low-income urban populations are: malaria, measles, tetanus, helminthic infestations, acute respiratory infections, diarrhoeal diseases, nutritional problems, communicable diseases other than those mentioned, and diseases of the skin. Among the adults, the main problems are: malaria, respiratory infections, pregnancy-related problems, hypertension, and diseases due to poor environmental hygiene and poor health habits.

There is a handful of special programmes for low-income urban groups. One of these is a government-planned programme in Etiosa (Lagos), which has a population of 158 000. Here a health clinic is run by the local government. A housing programme and road improvements are planned for the area. More health facilities, water works, a sewage treatment plant, and electricity are also to be provided for this complex of low-income groups. In addition, there are plans for an immunization programme and education in oral rehydration therapy.

The Lagos state government recently decided to upgrade some poor urban areas. Roads, piped water, markets, and schools would be provided "without necessarily disturbing the people".

Of the nongovernmental organizations, the Roman Catholic churches are developing ways of working among the urban poor. Their recent efforts are directed at slum areas. Their clinics are modest, but very strongly supported by outreach services. These are carried out by voluntary workers trained in simple but effective health skills and in the mobilization of the community for participation in health and other community development programmes.

An example of the universities' involvement with urban health care is a family health project started in a densely populated periurban area in Shomolu (Lagos). Run by the Institute of Child Health and Primary Care of the College of Medicine, University of Lagos, this has developed into a model project. Coverage is being "scaled up" from its present level (30 000 persons) to extend to the entire Shomolu local government area (population: 450 000), Few compounds in Shomolu have piped water, the other sources of water being wells or itinerant water-vendors. "Night-soil men" remove wastes from bucket latrines. There is electricity. There are few motorable roads, and so refuse trucks cannot reach the huge refuse dumps that make the area insanitary. Storm drains for floodwater in the rainy season are blocked by refuse. Agriculture is virtually non-existent in the area. In 1968 the crude birth rate was 62.8 per 1000, the crude death rate 14.1 per 1000, and the infant mortality rate 143 per 1000 live births.

No part of the target community is more than 10 minutes' walk from the clinic set up by the project. The target community includes many private medical facilities, both western and traditional—6 doctor's clinics, 2 hospitals with maternity wards, 25 traditional medical practitioners, 16 medicine stores, and 20 chemist's shops. Thus the area has been used to a very *ad hoc* approach to family health. The strong points of the project were that its facilities were accessible, acceptable, affordable, scientific, and evaluated, and that the approach adopted involved some community participation. Political changes have shifted the responsibility for the traditional systems of health care to the local government authorities, who do not always heed the wishes of the people. One criticism is that the clinic has not developed a system of referral to "higher" levels of health care.

A new "urban health problem" has recently emerged—the proliferation of mobile street traders. These young and energetic people sell their wares illegally to motorists and users of public transport caught in the frequent hold-ups and jams characteristic of traffic in Lagos. Programmes similar to those started for the "street children" in many Latin American cities may be appropriate here.

Prepared by Professor T. O. Johnson, Director, Institute of Child Health and Primary Care, College of Medicine, University of Lagos, Lagos, Nigeria.

Hospitals: the untapped resource

The concentration of curative facilities in large urban hospitals diverts resources from preventive services that are crucial for the health of the population. In most countries and cities, hospitals consume an extremely high proportion of the total health budget (as much as 80% in some cases). Too often they have little commitment to, or interest in, primary health care and play only a very limited role in helping to develop strategies and plans for it in the city. At the WHO/Aga Khan Foundation Conference on the Role of Hospitals in Primary Health Care (Karachi, November 1981) (62), Dr H. Mahler, the then Director-General of WHO, observed: "A health system based on primary health care cannot, and I repeat cannot be realized, cannot be developed, cannot function, and simply cannot exist without a network of hospitals with responsibility for supporting primary health care; promoting community health development action; basic and continuing education of all categories of health personnel; and research."

In fact, hospitals constitute a great untapped resource for the expansion of primary health care.

The conclusions of this Conference outlined a new and important role for the hospital, for which the prerequisites are (a) unambiguous support by political leaders and (b) appropriate guidance and coordination by government at each administrative level. Coordinating structures should include a committee, council, or board, where representatives for each part of the health system (hospitals, health centres, and primary care workers) can sit down with representatives of the community to deal with questions of policy, management, and resources. Every hospital should be associated with a well-defined catchment area within a district framework and should have a department of community health to mobilize interest, develop expertise, and interact with other health personnel inside and outside the hospital, and with the community in its catchment area.

The responsibilities of departments of community health should include: giving support and encouragement to primary health care in the catchment areas; providing in-service training to reorient hospital workers so that their "hospital outlook" is replaced by a "health outlook"; participating in the education and supervision of primary health care workers in the field; helping to improve management and administration; collaborating with the community in seeking relevant information on health problems and appropriate solutions; making sure that the hospital meets its responsibilities as regards referral and logistic support; developing effective ways in which the community can assist in improving hospital services; working with other public agencies, nongovernmental organizations, and community associations (including women's groups) active in the catchment area; identifying gaps in the primary health care services and introducing appropriate innovations; and stimulating

81

and conducting health services research focused on practical issues with the aim of achieving a progressive improvement in services.

The new Aga Khan Hospital and Medical College in Karachi is one teaching hospital that is consciously seeking to put these recommendations into practice, but there are other important examples, on which detailed information can be obtained from the International Hospital Federation.

The experience of the Aga Khan Health Services and Hospital in the context of primary health care in Karachi, Pakistan

In the early 1980s, the Aga Khan Health Services built and began to operate a 700-bed hospital in Karachi (Pakistan). The management committee and the supporters of the hospital were committed to ensuring that it developed, implemented, and maintained a primary health care programme. A major part of this commitment consisted in training professional health workers in the medical school attached to the hospital. The teaching programmes focus on field-oriented, community-based primary health care with priority for mothers and children, coupled with the control of endemic diseases. Students gain practical experience in the slums of Karachi, as well as in the very poor rural areas of the Sind and the northern frontier areas. Structurally the services for training new professional health workers in Karachi are divided into three tiers. These deal respectively with: (a) community health workers at the household and community level; (b) lady health visitors working from health posts to supervise the community health workers; and (c) doctor–nurse teams working from health centres to support groups (a) and (b). The referral system links the community with the base hospital, which is also committed to supporting primary health care. The training and orientation shared by both staff and students are beginning to show them the positive role hospitals can play in primary health care. It involves supporting community health needs, establishing role models for new medical staff, and enlisting the collaboration of other sectors in improving the health care of the very poor, especially in the urban slums.

In 1987, the WHO Expert Committee on the Role of Hospitals at the First Referral Level (63) stated that "currently, in most settings around the world, hospitals and the other local health services are not integrated. They are managed separately and their work is generally not well coordinated." The Expert Committee further asserted "that the conceptual focal point for organizational and functional integration should be the district health system encompassing the hospital and all other local health services".

This reorientation of the hospitals should facilitate and accompany the reorganization of the referral system within urban districts and a redistribution of the patient workload to permit a more efficient and coordinated use of all health facilities and make them more accessible (*64*).

A bold reorganization of this kind has been successfully attempted in Cali, Colombia (M. J. A. Escobar, unpublished information, 1979), in response to continually deteriorating conditions of overcrowding and improper utilization of central hospital facilities, and to the bypassing and underutilization of peripheral health units. This project was of particular benefit to poor populations living in peripheral *barrios*. In fact, one of its main achievements was the strengthening of peripheral facilities, thus removing the chief obstacle to their correct utilization and the main reason for overcrowding in the hospitals. By influencing the public through the mass media, religious and other organizations, and the schools, by making the home the basic service unit and by supplying professional health workers and medical students with relevant information, awareness on the part of those in the urban health system was improved, people were guided towards self-help and the appropriate use of health facilities, and feedback was encouraged. At the same time supportive supervision of the peripheral clinics and the logistics of their supply systems were revitalized.

Implementation

Policies, comprehensive health plans, and legislation are only as good as the commitment behind them, and the action that follows. In terms of implementation, almost everything remains to be done. The distribution of facilities and the financial and cultural constraints on access to services, are such that most poor people are patently underserved. Hospitals have traditionally been the main vehicles for the delivery of medical care to urban populations, but are generally at some remove, physically and socially, from the "new" urban poor. Moreover, the hospitals are already overcrowded, and their resources tightly stretched. There is a relative scarcity of more peripheral and accessible health and social services; where these exist, their quality may be so low that people are discouraged from using them.

If health administrations in the cities are unable to fulfil the essential requirements of the primary health care approach in an equitable and cost-effective manner, bringing multisectoral action to bear upon essential health needs, how likely are they to do so in the much more demanding situation of the rural areas? Yet the organization and functioning of health programmes in many urban districts leave much to be desired. A variety of ministries, social security organizations, municipal health departments, quasi-governmental organizations, and private institutions participate in these programmes. But these sources of action and influence, far from constituting a well-organized and synergistic network, often conflict with one another, duplicate activities and leave gaps in the programmes, struggle for funds and power, and produce an irrational and inefficient distribution of services. The results are high costs, dissatisfaction all round, and an inability to cope effectively with needs and demand.

Managing urban change

While, at present, natural increase probably accounts for at least 50% of urban growth in most cities, migration remains an important factor. As about two-thirds of migrants are in the age group 15–29 years, they create a demand for new employment opportunities that few cities are able to meet. Although migration is usually considered to impose social costs, this is not always so and, in many cases, it may benefit cities' economies. Migrants often work in "informal sectors" and fulfil important functions.

The impact of migration is uneven and now it is generally the outer fringes of the cities that have become the foci of urban growth. The large metropolitan areas have tended to lose their predominance, experiencing some decline in population, jobs, and services. This is a problem that is also increasingly affecting older suburbs and some overspill towns.

Against this background, one obvious question is whether and how further immigration should be resisted. Many methods have been tried, such as:

- a system of identity cards and residence permits, enforced with police support, and physical clearance of illegal settlements (these were the policies until recently in Nairobi and Khartoum);

- policies and projects for rural regeneration (as in the United Republic of Tanzania);

- decentralization of industry to encourage population growth away from the main conurbation (as in Indonesia);

- incentives, such as free or subsidized land and loans for construction, to encourage people to settle where the government thinks that they should—as in Juba (Sudan) and, most recently, in Pakistan.

The available evidence suggests that none of these methods works particularly well. Several countries (e.g., Indonesia and Mozambique) have now accepted this fact and are not resisting *ad hoc* settlements. They are, however, encouraging traditional forms of mutual self-help.

It goes almost without saying that, once continuing immigration is accepted, along with recognition of past illegal immigration, there is no escaping some formidable management dilemmas in areas ranging from policing and welfare functions to the promotion and encouragement of development activities.

Maputo, Mozambique

As elsewhere in Africa, the major source of urban growth in Mozambique is the rapid influx to the city of migrants from rural areas (accounting for 66% of urban population growth), rather than natural increase. Maputo had about one million inhabitants in 1985 and an annual growth rate of 8%. Migrants from the countryside usually move into the homes of relatives in Maputo, which increases overcrowding and facilitates the transmission of infectious and parasitic diseases. Environmental hygiene becomes a particular problem in these circumstances. The City Council is trying to tackle this problem by creating new "wards" (areas) which are provided with building plots and services. Here, people build their own homes and have land on which to grow food, while the population density is about 70 per hectare.

Various integrated health projects have been started in these peripheral areas. An example is the Joint WHO/UNICEF Nutrition Support Programme financed by the Government of Italy. The emphasis on agriculture and health and social issues in this programme has improved the nutritional status of children in the areas. The City Health Directorate has also received support from nongovernmental organizations, particularly religious groups.

Intersectoral coordination is facilitated by the mass democratic organizations (including women's and youth organizations), "action groups" at neighbourhood level (typically with different individuals responsible for health, education, food supply, etc.), the City Party Committee, and the City Council. Support from the Ministry of Health is mainly limited to evaluation at the national level and thus is not concerned with specific health problems in the city.

The particular health problems currently faced in the city reflect the fact that the country is at war. The low-income population makes up about 30% of the total urban population, and most of its members are unemployed, having recently migrated from the rural areas. Malaria has been a particular problem and, in the field of sanitation, efforts are being made to increase the construction of latrines and the drainage of mosquito breeding-places. There have also been considerable improvements in the water supply programme.

Until 1980, Maputo recorded epidemic outbreaks of measles every 2 years with as many as 1500 cases per month and a high fatality rate. Vaccination coverage has been increased, and now the annual incidence is 200–300 cases per 100 000 population with no peaks.

The incidence of diarrhoeal diseases is still very high. Fortunately most infants are breast-fed, but diarrhoeal diseases occur with the introduction of other types of food and worsen during the weaning period. Poor environmental hygiene and overcrowding contribute to this situation. It is thought that the transmission of disease is not through water but person-to-person. The use of oral rehydration therapy is slowly increasing.

Acute respiratory infections are important from June onwards when they take precedence over malaria and diarrhoea. Again, it is the children who are the worst affected, and overcrowding exacerbates the problem. There are no programmes to deal with the situation, as it has not been studied epidemiologically and a strategy has thus not been worked out.

The overall annual incidence of tuberculosis in Maputo is 250 per 100 000, and its prevalence almost 600 per 100 000. A big problem is that of patients abandoning treatment. Often they turn first to traditional healers for help, so that proper diagnosis is delayed.

Neonatal tetanus in children has been successfully controlled by immunization programmes.

Over 60% of the population are infested by *Ascaris*, but the latrine-building programmes in peripheral areas will help to reduce this problem.

Injuries resulting from road accidents are common; these are often associated with alcohol abuse. Among domestic accidents, burns are important, while, following the installation of people from rural areas in multistorey buildings after independence, there was a great increase in the number of children killed by falling from windows or balconies.

Ninety per cent of the children born in Maputo in 1985 had a birth-weight of over 2.5 kg. However, in the poorer groups an appreciable number of children have a low weight-for-age. The proportion is less than 10% in the first year of life, more than 20% in the second year of life, and about 20% in the third, dropping to between 10% and 15% in the fourth year. With an economic situation that precludes the import of needed food items and a war that curtails agricultural activities, the nutritional problem is serious and is attracting the attention of various international agencies.

Maputo has 16 health centres, 40 health posts, and 6 hospitals. There is an urgent need for health centres in the new "wards". At the moment the residents in these poverty-stricken new peripheral settlements have very long distances to travel. Resources are in short supply, particularly drugs. It is hoped that the introduction of an essential drugs programme will ease the situation. However, the future looks problematic and there is a feeling in the health sector that ground is being lost.

Prepared by Dr Campos José Maria de Igrejas, Director of Health, Maputo City.

Chapter 3

Community involvement

Linking health systems and communities

As a number of countries, notably China (65), have shown, people's potential for improving their own health and living conditions is enormous. When the community is fully involved, collaboration between different sectors is often greatly simplified. Indeed it is not overstating the case to say that community involvement is essential for health development (66). Nevertheless, it usually remains very limited in the numerous countries where planning, priority-setting, and implementation are left to health service staff, while the people for whom health services are intended seem to have little say in the matter.

With strong community organization, a well-informed local health committee capable of assuming responsibility, and logistic support, a large measure of decentralization and delegation becomes feasible.

Neighbourhood health programmes are a valuable means of increasing primary health care in urban districts. There is no established blueprint for them, since their nature will vary according to local conditions. Different models exist in different cities, and more are being developed. Sometimes an approach successfully initiated in the countryside and based on family spirit and solidarity has later been adapted to specific urban settings. This is the case of the *kebele*, *barrio*, and *kampung* community health development schemes of, respectively, Addis Ababa, Cali (Colombia) and Jakarta. Others were urban schemes from the start. The *barangay* development programme of Manila is a good example. Its main features, which are common to other, similar programmes, include: a close knowledge of the community, the prevention and treatment of malnutrition, immunization, the treatment of easily recognizable diseases, referral systems, environmental improvements and information and education for the families concerned. The programme is

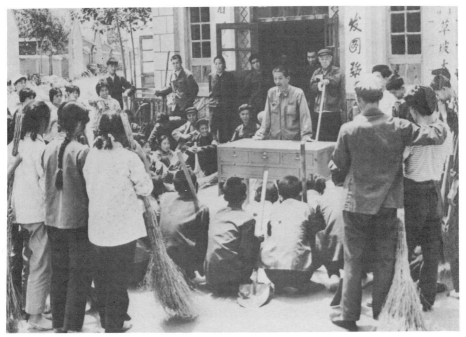

WHO/Ministry of Public Health, China (19492)

Community involvement in China has led to significant improvements in health and living conditions

based in the community health centre, the upgrading of which is continually pursued. It emphasizes the training and wide deployment of community health workers and the education of the public by all available means.

Women have a fundamental role in community health, being at the same time the protagonists and one of the main target groups. They are close to the children, the most vulnerable group of the population, at the most critical moments of their lives; they are closely involved in and affected by decisions on contraception, on breast-feeding, and on the quality of their children's food. They may tip the balance in the prevention of disease, and it is they who will most probably have to decide what to do and whom to consult when a child is sick. They keep "urban gardens", when there is space for them, and raise poultry or small animals. Economically, it is they who have to make ends meet in the family, who are the heads of most single-parent households, and who earn needed supplementary income. They benefit from, but also run, the community crèches and the day-care centres for preschool children. They are without doubt those in whom money for education is best invested.

C. A. Frankenhoff (unpublished observations, 1976) notes that ". . . it is essential to facilitate the involvement of untapped resources of marginal communities into the process of urban development". There are political, social, and economic arguments in favour of this option. "The political argument states that increasing the stability of these slum communities in terms of jobs, housing, education and health will contribute to national political stability. The social argument states that the community which has helped to build itself will produce social benefits for the nation. The economic argument states that the slum community can generate significant consumer demands as well as capital formation. Houses, sewers, sidewalks, schools and clinics can be built by such a community with a minimum of assistance."

The initiative and resourcefulness of low-income urban populations are increasingly recognized by planners and other government officials. There is of course a danger that overemphasis on community action may be used as a pretext for withholding government support, but experience has shown that in practice neither the exclusively community-managed self-help programme, nor the paternalistic government-sponsored and imposed community programme, is an ideal solution. Success is more likely to occur when a partnership between government and community is established, entailing recognition of what self-help can do, respect for the individual, and willingness on the part of the authorities to go along with community initiatives (67).

A UNICEF review (68), based on information from 70 countries, including case studies from 9 of them, concluded that the community-based approach is viable and is being increasingly adopted. It enables services to reach out further towards the poorest families; to be designed in direct response to needs that the people themselves have expressed and thus to be better understood and supported; to be more highly valued and better maintained by the community; and to be relatively inexpensive, while permitting increased coverage. By encouraging social action, this approach helps to promote social cohesion as well.

There are different methods of implementing the partnership mentioned above (69, 70) but these do not lend themselves to any simple classification. Success is more likely when the community has a clear understanding of the problems being faced, and when initiatives come from within it .

Developments that are the result of a true dialogue between government and communities, with mutual acknowledgement of the contributions made by each, are few and far between. The community development scheme in Ricinha (Rio de Janeiro) (*71*) is a possible example. The residents formed a health group, a sanitation group, and a school group, and worked together with the municipal secretariat for social development, first on a survey and then on the planning of a programme based on the survey. The resulting activities included child and adult education, a sanitation programme, and the provision of health services. The main sewer system was established through mutual help, and secondary connections were built by the community. Community agents have been trained to monitor growth in children under 5 years of age and to help form women's health education groups. The programme and its methodology have been institutionalized, and expansion to other areas is being considered.

Then there is the example of the creation of community kitchens in Kamanves, a slum in Miraj, India (*72*). This was initially part of a comprehensive effort to improve the nutritional status of the population, and was later developed well beyond its original objectives. Following a discussion of local problems in the community, a group of residents formed a committee, which, after consultation with the Director of Community Health, started to work with hospital staff in a series of activities involving all community residents. An organization was established, a management committee was elected, and fees were collected from all members. The first initiative was a morning feeding programme for children, later expanded to cover very poor adults at a cost of 0.60 rupees per person. The kitchen, which was initially uncovered, was later provided with a shelter. The children attending were medically examined. The programme was expanded to include training and income-generating activities. The health education programme was particularly important and led, among other things, to high rates of immunization with diphtheria-pertussis-tetanus, poliomyelitis, smallpox, and tuberculosis (BCG) vaccines.

Local organizations for community involvement

In rural areas, community organization is often based on solid social and cultural foundations and has developed over centuries. It remains reasonably efficient and is largely taken for granted. All this is lost with migration to the cities, and the delicate tissue of social organization has somehow to be woven anew.

Yet the conditions needed to redevelop social organization are difficult to establish. In the new slums and squatter settlements, little

91

is generally done to guide rural migrants through the transition from rural to urban life.

In contrast to the relatively stable and homogeneous rural village, these migrants are likely to find themselves in a society that is heterogeneous, both culturally and linguistically, transient, mobile, opportunistic and restless, with each person too preoccupied with his or her individual survival to be concerned with solving collective problems.

While these are divisive features, some people nevertheless feel united by the fact that they inhabit the same place and share poverty and pressing common problems to which some solution must be found. It is "neighbourhood awareness", called by different names in different places, that provides the main basis for the social organization of the urban poor and thus for some improvement in their living conditions.

One purpose of community development is to enable people living in the poorest areas to gain organizational and managerial experience and confidence in dealing with government and other organizations, and in building up mechanisms that demand responsibility and accountability on the part of those providing resources as well as the community. Nylon, a periurban slum area near the airport of Douala, Cameroon, is a good example of how this process can develop and enable community goals to be met by the residents (73). Nylon is a slum which was estimated to have reached a population of more than 100 000 by 1980, yet, until a few years ago, the area was marked on city maps as an uninhabited zone, so that the population had no legal existence. Initially, the three ethnic groups living in Nylon decided to join in a common effort to fight water pollution, industrial pollution, and growing vandalism. The area was divided into lots, blocks, sectors, and subdivisions, and "animators"—each accountable to the corresponding person at the next higher level—were assigned to each unit. The leaders then sought municipal assistance, organized a seminar on the urban environment, which drew public attention to their problems, and established a training programme for the animators. Official recognition was obtained from the Ministry of Social Affairs, and a community centre was constructed. Later, a topographical survey was carried out, and a master plan for development drawn up. Electricity was installed and, with foreign aid, work started on the construction of a new market-place. Community activities in Nylon gave rise to the concept of a "transitional urban economy", which is neither traditional nor modern, being characterized by a predominance of "unemployed" persons among the workers in the informal sector, simple methods of production, and a complex network of ties with the modern economic sector, whose by-products and waste materials are exploited to the maximum. Since self-sufficiency in food is considered to be a prerequisite of the transitional urban economy, all available land was intensively cultivated, poultry was raised, and a small-scale food industry was started as an experiment.

Many cities in the developing world have evolved some forms of local organization encouraging community involvement. To take only a few examples:

- In Indonesia, the "Community Resilience Boards" act as bridges between government and community. These boards, which exist all over the country, have a variety of sections, including health sections.

- In Pakistan, elected local bodies form committees for various purposes. The health committees (including, for example, mullahs, teachers, and elders) provide a link between the health authorities and local communities.

- In Mozambique, the pattern of community organization is basically very much the same as in Indonesia, with a village-level set-up supplemented by neighbourhood and block associations.

- In Colombia, there are, in the big cities, Community Action Boards similar to the Community Resilience Boards in Indonesia. These are organizations of the urban poor and are strong because they are rooted in their communities, but their health component is relatively weak.

- In Manila and other cities in the Philippines, the *Barangay* Council is the political body at the neighbourhood level for population units of 2000 or thereabouts. The Council is supplemented by a *barangay* network consisting of, among others, *purok* and unit leaders, volunteers (including health workers), and sometimes representatives of nongovernmental organizations. Religious bodies may also form committees to deal with selected aspects of primary health care.

- In Juba (Sudan), there are "Quarter Councils", which elect representatives to the municipality. Health is one of their interests. Initiatives are passed down from the Ministry of Health to the councillors, then down to the different communities. The feedback from each community indicates whether it is enthusiastic about taking ideas further. If there is a positive response, a community committee will pursue the matter.

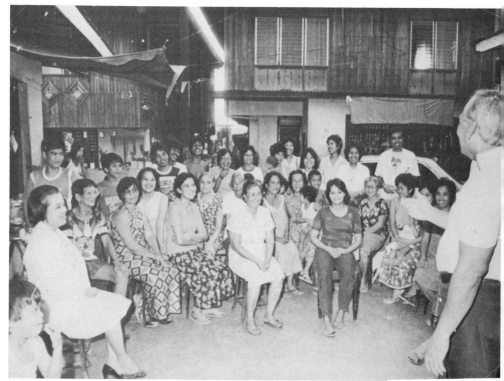

WHO/E. Suva (19108)

A *barangay* meeting in Manila allows discussion of the community's health care problems and priorities

- In Somalia, there are community organizations (known as *tabella*) in all cities, each covering 50–100 families. The *tabella*-level committee, whose members are chosen by the local community and are unpaid, is responsible for all communal activities within the *tabella* and has full executive authority.

- In Thai cities, not all communities have recognized organizations. Where these do exist, community health workers may be attached to them to promote primary health care. Otherwise, as community health workers are trained, special committees have to be set up to provide a focal point for their activities.

Many other examples could be cited. These, however, do give a small idea of the range of community organizations, which extends from some that are strong and well accepted to some that are quite weak; from some that cover the whole of a community's interests to

94

some that are health-specific; from some that are seen as useful for consultation to some that are absolutely vital to health; and from some that are truly representative of a particular community to some that are primarily instruments of government. While different organizations are acceptable in different social and political contexts, primary health care calls for strong local neighbourhood organizations with a genuine degree of interdependence of action and autonomy of choice and preferably covering all sectors, not just health.

The situation in Merka City, Somalia

Primary health care activities in Somalia began in 1981. Programmes are in operation in 8 out of 18 regions and are assisted by various international, bilateral and nongovernmental bodies including the Government of Italy, USAID, UNICEF, WHO, and CARITAS.

No figures are available on the extent of the low-income urban population in the country, but it is thought that their main health problems are diarrhoeal diseases, pneumonia, malnutrition, anaemia, and bronchitis. Action being taken to overcome these problems includes water and sanitation programmes, "family life education", control of diarrhoeal diseases, and the extension of maternal and child health services. The main problems are a lack of manpower and a shortage of funds.

In Merka (near Mogadishu, the capital) slum dwellers form the majority of the population. The main health problems of the city as a whole are the lack of an adequate supply of safe drinking-water and the absence of proper facilities for refuse and excreta disposal. About 50% of the low-income population are considered to be adequately covered by primary health care at present.

Special funds for the region in which the city is situated have been allocated by the Joint WHO/UNICEF Nutrition Support Programme. Only 5.8% of the Ministry of Health's budget is earmarked for primary health care, and there are difficulties in shifting additional financial resources away from prestige facilities, such as hospitals.

Community participation is fostered through regular meetings with committee leaders who select community health workers and traditional birth attendants for training and subsequently supervise them. It is felt that the communities could take a more active part in primary health care by organizing environmental sanitation compaigns, thus compensating for the shortage of health manpower.

An understanding of the needs of the urban poor can only be achieved when the health information system in Somalia is improved. At present it is very poor in terms of vital statistics and demographic and health indicators. Data collected since 1984 indicate that the main causes of mortality and morbidity in Merka are as follows:

Main causes of death by age group:
under 1 year: diarrhoea, respiratory infections, neonatal causes, malnutrition;
1–4 years: diarrhoea, respiratory infections, measles, malnutrition;
5–14 years: measles, diarrhoea;
15–44 years: measles;
over 45 years: tuberculosis, malaria, gastrointestinal diseases.

Main reasons for admission to hospital by age group:
under 1 year: respiratory infections, diarrhoea;
1–4 years: respiratory infections, diarrhoea;
5–14 years: tuberculosis;
15–44 years: malaria;
over 45 years: malaria.

Prepared by Dr G. M. Dini, Regional Primary Health Care Coordinator, Lower Shabelle Region, Ministry of Health, Somalia.

There are also failures, as might be expected, for the circumstances of the urban poor make success more surprising than failure. People in long-established slums often experience more difficulty in working together for the common well-being than those in new slums and squatter areas. There is a sense of inertia, and substantial doubts about whether collective action is possible or worth the trouble. The main constraints lie with the poor themselves, who rarely have the social confidence, skills, and experience to galvanize their own community, deal collectively with government officials and nongovernmental organizations, and, if the need arises, challenge other people's hostile attitudes and actions.

Government collaboration with communities may be hampered by excessively technical approaches, inadequate mechanisms for social planning, an insistence on technical standards that are unrealistic and unnecessarily high, inappropriate legislation, administrative bottlenecks, and an inability of officials to communicate with the community and to understand the dynamics of an urban slum (*74*).

96

Likewise, nongovernmental organizations may define health programmes in terms of their own perceptions, pursue short-term goals, and unintentionally create dependent attitudes that are not conducive to community initiative, organization, and action.

The role of facilitators

Where strong community organizations do not exist in poor urban neighbourhoods, they need to be created. This can be a long, complex, and difficult process, and an organizer usually has to be brought in from the outside. This organizer must be well trained and have the knowledge and skills required to analyse the social structure of the community, and to facilitate the participation of the people themselves in the organizational process. The essential steps in organizing communities are:

1. to develop enough initial understanding and trust to warrant the effort involved on the part of the community and the external staff, and to try to avoid disappointing the community;

2. to conduct a baseline survey and a social analysis: this could be done with the help of a university-based research team and should involve the community;

3. to continue to build up a rapport with the community, while analyses are being completed;

4. to hold discussions with members of the community to find out what are considered to be the most pressing problems faced by the community as a whole. In these discussions, the community organizer should provide feedback on the results of the baseline survey to corroborate people's identification of priority problems, or to show them that other problems are equally important. The ultimate aim of these discussions is to obtain a consensus on a feasible starting-point for action by the community. This could take the form of the construction (on a self-help basis) of solid walkways, as in Olongapo (Philippines); the provision of subsidized meals for street children; educational work among squatter or immigrant children, as in Hong Kong; shelter improvement, as in Nairobi; or low-cost self-help housing as in Hyderabad, Visakhapatnam, and many other Indian cities. The initial project need not necessarily be connected with primary health care in a narrow sense. It is a springboard for organized community action which, if it achieves results, will motivate community members to deal with a wider range of development activities in similar fashion.

The community organizers could be the health staff, as in Jakarta and Manila, or the community development staff of an agency like the Department of Social Services, as in Nairobi. The community organizer could come from a nongovernmental organization, as in the case of Olongapo City (Philippines) or the Kwun Tong Project in Hong Kong. It is important to stress that health officers taking on the role of community organizer must be thoroughly trained for it. Otherwise they will quickly find themselves out of their depth, and the resulting organization may simply cater to the interests of the vocal and relatively better-off minority, to the neglect of poorer groups.

Community involvement in an Indian city

Visakhapatnam had a total of 800 000 inhabitants in 1986, a quarter of whom were living in slums. Reliable information is available on the health situation in the slum areas, which is substantially worse than that in the city as a whole. For example, 20% of children under 5 years old in the poorer areas are severely malnourished, compared with a city average of 10%.

The main communicable diseases in the city are tuberculosis, gastroenteritis, worm infestation, viral hepatitis A, malaria, skin diseases, sexually transmitted diseases, and leprosy. The prevalence of these diseases is about 25% higher in the slums than in other areas of the city.

At present about 50% of the slum population is covered by primary health care, the principal agency involved being the municipal corporation.

The urban community development project (in operation since 1981) aims to provide an integrated package of basic services to urban slum-dwellers. This comprises: (a) basic amenities, such as water supply and sanitation; (b) health services, particularly immunization, oral rehydration therapy, and maternal and child health care; (c) basic education services (including preschool and adult education); (d) leadership training programmes covering the identification and resolution of community problems; (e) income-generating programmes for poor women; and (f) programmes to enhance the planning and implementation capacities of the project and of the municipal corporation.

The project has created multipurpose workers known as community organizers and social workers. There is one organizer or social worker for every 3–4 slums (approximately 3000 people). Refresher courses are held every year and the community organizers and social workers train community leaders, mothers, unemployed young people, and others.

Following the principle that the community must find solutions to its own problems, other features of the programme include:

— the creation of neighbourhood funds, including grants from the urban community development project, and the opening of a bank account;

— joint management of funds by the president of the neighbourhood committee and the community organizers and social workers;

— the organization and running of preschool and craft centres, training classes, educational campaigns, and immunization and oral rehydration therapy programmes, through neighbourhood committees;

— regular meetings of neighbourhood committee members, attended by community organizers, social workers, and voluntary workers;

— bringing the clinics' problems to the notice of the municipal authorities through neighbourhood committees, and solving them;

— low-cost, self-help housing with loans from the municipality and banks, government subsidies, and contributions from the beneficiaries (by now, about 7200 dwellings housing 40 000 slum-dwellers have been completed, at a cost of US$ 1000 per house);

— low-cost sanitation: conversion of dry-earth latrines to low-cost pour-flush latrines and provision of latrines to households lacking them. The cost of each latrine is $100 (provided on a 50% loan and 50% subsidy basis); so far, about 5000 have been installed.

Another interesting project run by the municipality is the "social forestry" scheme. Nineteen thousand plants have been set on road verges and wasteland. Women, former leprosy patients, and physically handicapped persons have been chosen to look after them. Each is responsible for between 100 and 200 plants and is given a plot near the plants on which to erect a dwelling and a stall where he or she can sell tea, matches, cigarettes, etc. The municipality pays 2 rupees a month for every surviving plant. Ninety people are involved so far, and the plant survival rate is 99%.

Major problems still to be dealt with include: the lack of a clear health plan for the city, the relatively low priority given to health, and the very high cost of improving the urban infrastructure.

Prepared by Mr P. K. Mohanty, Commissioner, Municipal Commission, Visakhapatnam, India.

Community health workers

The generic term "community health worker" includes a very wide variety of health personnel. Depending on the country, they may be: paid or voluntary; male or female; young or mature; full-time or part-time; trained for as little as 1–2 weeks or for as long as a year; and expected to serve as few as 50 or as many as 4000 people.

In most parts of the world, community health workers constitute the foundation of primary health care in urban areas. Linking the community with the health system, they have loyalties to both (Fig. 8).

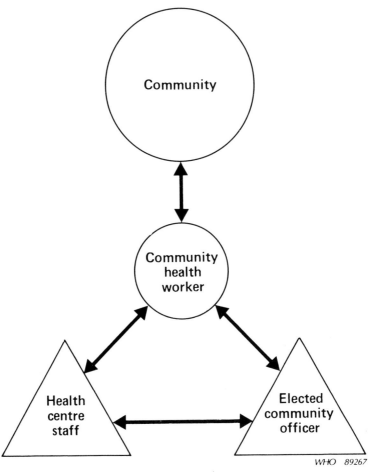

Fig. 8. Community health workers: the bridge between communities and the health system

The community health worker is one of the principal figures in neighbourhood health development, meeting the need for close contact with the community, emphasizing health promotion and disease prevention rather than strictly curative medicine, and paying special attention to people's behaviour and the environment in which they live. This approach is also a way of compensating for the scarcity of professional health workers, whether this scarcity is real or due to their inequitable distribution or reluctance to work in poor areas. It is accepted in several cities as a means of filling the gaps in services.

Because of the greater availability of facilities for treatment in urban areas, community health workers are primarily concerned with health promotion, disease prevention, and the orientation of the public to a better utilization of the health system. They visit people in their homes and so are able to assess the social and environmental conditions in which they live, and to act as a link between the public and the health system, the user and the provider of health services. However, the deployment of community health workers and, in particular, their participation in the diagnosis and treatment of some diseases, has aroused greater opposition among professional health workers in the cities than among their rural counterparts. Also, to work unpaid or be paid in kind is not feasible for long in a city, and the turnover among such workers tends to be high. In spite of these difficulties, where community health workers exist, they provide a vital service.

It is essential that the community health worker should truly belong to the community concerned, through living in it and being accountable to it.

Community health workers should evolve in line with needs. Their programmes should be reviewed regularly and should not impose so heavy a workload that the workers are unable to think critically about their tasks. Continuous training is required, and it should, to some extent, be left to the discretion of the experienced worker to use time as she or he judges best. Community health workers need to collaborate closely with others outside the formal health system and to become outspoken advocates for the community when health is at risk. The formal health system must stand behind them in such circumstances, even though this may require courage.

Since the community health worker is a link between the formal health service on the one hand and the community on the other, careful arrangements are needed to ensure that the selection, remuneration, and continuing supervision of community health workers are carried out jointly by the community and the formal health service in a genuine spirit of partnership. It may require a significant change of attitude by those in charge of the formal health system to accept that the community concerned should have this degree of control over community health workers.

The method for nomination or preselection of candidates is crucial and should reflect the type of participation that is appropriate to the particular community. If the community concerned does not participate in the selection process, the personality of the first-line worker is all the more important, for she or he must then win and retain the community's confidence.

Community health workers must keep records on the families they serve. The decision as to which information is passed back up the system, and what comes down through it, needs very careful thought. Otherwise, once again, the health system will collect data of little use and have no way of judging what needs to be known about health needs and the effectiveness of health action.

Some community health workers may wish to gain formal health credentials, and they should be helped to do so. If they have to leave their community for this purpose, they will need to be replaced, since their relationship with the community will inevitably be changed as a result.

A recent report of a study in which 11 countries took part discusses a number of relevant issues (75). While it is based on experience in the use of community health workers in rural areas, many of its conclusions are equally applicable in an urban context.

In principle, it is right that the community should select its own community health workers, but unfortunately this may sometimes be done before either the community or its leaders have acquired any real understanding of what a primary health care programme involves, and what a community health worker is supposed to do. If health centre staff can prepare people appropriately beforehand, selection may be improved and subsequent difficulties avoided.

What should be the role of community health workers? A common error is to ask too much of them. To make undue demands on a health worker, who may have a limited educational background and has received only a few weeks training, is to ask for trouble, especially with part-time workers. In the 11-country study on community health workers, referred to above, 22 different health tasks were listed in the job descriptions cited. Eight countries also required their community health workers to do work entirely outside the health sector. The medicines at the disposal of health workers for distribution or sale varied widely in type and number, ranging from 6 items in one country to over 70 in another.

Community health workers in Lima, Peru

Metropolitan Lima has about 5.2 million inhabitants (1981 census) of whom 2.7 million, representing 51% of the total population, live in marginal low-income areas.

A variety of projects are in progress, covering approximately 25% of the low-income population so far. They include promotional and preventive services addressed to individuals (e.g., education of mothers during examination and immunization of their children) and groups: first aid, the treatment of major diseases, and the follow-up of treatment previously prescribed. Other government sectors, such as education and labour, make various contributions to family welfare, for example, through activities to promote the development of preschool children (3–5 years) and the advancement of women including training in ways of improving the family income, etc.

Community health workers of two different types (promoters and secretaries) participate in health promotion and preventive work, education, surveillance, and welfare. They are selected by the community to which they are accountable, and trained by the health teams at government health centres. They are assigned to the "modules" into which the area is divided (so far 65 modules have been established), each worker being responsible for 10–25 families (generally 100 families are covered by a health promoter and 4 health secretaries). The work is voluntary and unpaid.

The training of community health workers forms an important part of the projects. The promoters are given a month's training in theory and practical work leading to a general qualification, while two months' additional training is required for specific qualifications in certain areas according to the needs of the community. Continuing in-service training follows.

Comparing the present situation with that obtaining before the projects, improvements can be noted in health awareness, nutritional status, immunization coverage, drinking-water supplies (present coverage, 80%), garbage collection (present coverage, 20%), and school attendance.

The projects are financed by the government, local communities, and UNICEF. There is active coordination with other sectors according to situations and needs; with local authorities (municipalities) to plan activities jointly, avoiding duplication and benefiting from mutual support; with private institutions; and with other projects having similar objectives.

Prepared by Dr Oscar Castillo, Primary Health Care Consultant to UNICEF, Lima, Peru.

Table 5. Data on community health workers in various countries and territories

City and/or country	Type of worker[a]	No. of families (or localities) per worker	Paid	Working hours	Type of care[b]	Training	Sex
Bangkok, Thailand	Peri-urban: VHV	100–150	no	irregular	P/C	2 or more weeks	M/F
	VHC Congested areas:	10–15	no	irregular	P	1 week	M/F
	UHV	15–25	no	irregular	P/C	2 weeks	M/F
Bogotá, Colombia		50	no	3	P/C	30 hours	M/F
Cebu, Philippines		20	no	3	P/C	6 weeks	F
Hong Kong	CHW	varies with area	yes	full-time	P/C	about 6 months	M/F
	CHV	varies with area	no	part-time	P/C	from 6 weeks	M/F
India		20–25	no	part-time	P	2 weeks+ refresher	M/F
Jakarta/Surabaya, Indonesia		50	no	3	P/C	2 weeks	M/F
Juba, Sudan		(a) 100+	yes	full-time	P/C+ immunization	9 months	M
		(b) ?	no	2	P	6 weeks	F
Lagos, Nigeria		(a) 150–200	yes	full-time	P/C	9 months	M/F
		(b) 50	no	irregular	P	3 weeks	M/F

Manila, Philippines	barangay health volunteers 10–20	no	irregular	P/C	2 weeks?	M/F
Maputo, Mozambique	(a) 50 houses	no	part-time	P	Continuous in reunions (no course)	M/F
	(b) 10 families	no	part-time	P		M/F
Nairobi, Kenya	39	no	irregular	P		M/F
Olongapo, Philippinés	50	no	full-time	P/C	27 days 120 hours	M/F
Pakistan	one village 200–300 people	no	part-time	P/C	12 weeks	M/F
Philippines (nongovernmental)	20–25	no	full-time	P/C	15–20 days staggered	M/F
Shanghai, China	500–600	yes	full-time	P/C	6 months	M/F
Somalia	300–400	no	full-time	P/C	6 weeks	M/F
Sri Lanka	50–60	no	part-time	P	1 week + refresher	M/F

[a] VHV: village health volunteer; VHC: village health coordinator; UHV: urban health volunteer; CHW: community health worker; CHV: community health volunteer.
[b] P: preventive; C: simple curative.

105

Despite differences in the duration, content, and level of training, certain general principles may be derived from experience in the countries taking part in the study. As far as possible, preservice training should be spaced out over several courses. Though relatively costly, this system is particularly effective.

In-service training should be continuous and is crucial for maintaining the motivation and competence of volunteers. In some places, e.g. Bangkok, Colombia, and Manila, self-learning manuals are used for training and for reference. Community leaders may also undergo orientation to primary health care and leadership training, as in Bangkok, Manila, Nairobi, and throughout Indonesia. In Visakhapatnam, India, the mayor and city councillors receive similar training. Courses in financial management may also be provided for volunteers, as in Manila and Thailand, where health insurance and credit unions are among the subjects covered.

The teaching method most commonly employed, namely lecturing, is often the least suitable. A variety of methods should be encouraged: discussion, demonstrations, supervised practical work, field visits, role-playing, and self-learning exercises. It is important to teach the trainees not only what to teach but how to teach it.

The supervision of community health workers is a major problem. In theory, it would be an advantage if the instructor during training could also be the supervisor afterwards. In practice, difficulties have arisen where this has been attempted. Supervision is not a popular activity, even with the supervisors themselves, for many of whom it simply means additional work and responsibility without reward or recognition, and without the training in management that they need.

Thus, the question of incentives is as relevant for supervisors as it is for community health workers. Job satisfaction, moral support, and acceptance by the community are even greater incentives than economic reward. Hence, the importance of adequate social preparation of the community and its leaders.

It is important for community health workers to have clearly defined roles. In India, for example, they often have written descriptions of their roles and a code of ethics. Their main functions are likely to be preventive—for example, monitoring health conditions and services in their community; giving advice on nutrition, hygiene, and health care; and recording data. They may also have curative functions (besides the administration of basic first aid), but these need to be carefully chosen in the light of their own skills and the functions of others, including the professional health workers.

In all the cities under review, volunteers have been nominated by community leaders, as in Jakarta and Manila, or elected by the

106

people as in Olongapo (Philippines), to facilitate effective community participation in health activities. The following are typical steps in the selection and training of volunteer community health workers.

1. Decide with the community on the criteria for selecting community health workers.

2. Select community health workers according to the agreed criteria.

3. Train the selected workers in:

    (*a*) community organization;
    (*b*) health care;
    (*c*) effective sharing of knowledge and skills;
    (*d*) group discussion; and
    (*e*) leadership.

4. Continue their development, using statistical and other data, their own knowledge, technical advice from professional health staff, and community views to redefine roles and targets.

5. Carry out training of community health workers in the development of simple managerial skills on a continuing basis.

Examples of community involvement

Each of the cities under review has involved communities in preliminary survey work and has some type of ongoing health information system. However, two examples are particularly impressive. The information system in Manila, which is based on growth charts kept in homes and notebooks kept by volunteers, seems to have been very effective. The amount of information collected is kept to the minimum needed and is simple enough to permit analysis and use at the community level. The "basic minimum needs" community survey and information system, recently introduced in Bangkok, measures 33 indicators of overall development and compares these indicators with target levels. Thus, it not only provides a baseline of household and community information, but also identifies the specific households and sectors where improvements are needed. The health indicators employed include: prevalence of malnutrition, immunization coverage, water and sanitation facilities, acceptance of family planning, utilization of maternal and child health services, some morbidity indicators, and the number of infants with low birth weight. These indicators are set in a much broader context of overall development (see Annex 1).

Most cities and countries seem to have introduced community-based growth monitoring through periodic weighing. In Thailand, weighings are performed every 3 months for normal children and more frequently for those suffering from malnutrition. In Indonesia and Mozambique combined growth monitoring, maternal and child health, and immunization services are provided on a monthly basis. Indonesia's impressive "five tables" system (see Table 6) is based on a network of integrated community health posts. Monthly weighings are included in Manila's primary health care programme. In the Philippines, growth monitoring is combined with nutrition education in most cases, and with supplementary feeding where there is second- and third-degree malnutrition.

Table 6. Indonesia's "five tables" system based on integrated community health posts

Table	Activity	Done by:
I	registration	volunteers
II	weighing of under-fives	volunteers
III	interpretation of growth chart	volunteers
	health education	volunteers
IV	distribution of contraceptives	volunteers
	distribution of drugs (including vitamins, iron tablets, oral rehydration salts, etc.)	volunteers
	first aid/simple treatment	volunteers
V	examination of pregnant women	health centre
	immunization	staff helped by the volunteers
	Special examinations of persons referred to health centres by the volunteers	

Support to enable communities to help themselves

All the countries with effective arrangements for community health workers provide some type of health kit to volunteers, along with educational materials, growth charts, scales, and other minor equipment. Articles such as radios, bicycles, public address systems (Thailand), and uniforms (Manila) are also considered as incentives for health workers, whether paid or volunteers. Other incentives include free medical care in most countries, subsidized basic commodities in the Philippines, and study tours to other communities or cities.

Support through the media seems common: films are used widely in Mozambique, a volunteers' newsletter in Thailand, and radio and television in the Philippines and Thailand.

Direct grants to communities for establishing certain kinds of activity are also an important form of support. Thailand provides grants as seed capital for the establishment of drug cooperatives, a revolving fund for the improvement of sanitation, and funds to improve nutrition. In Manila, seed money is provided (often by civic organizations such as Lions or Rotary Clubs) to establish a credit union/health insurance scheme and to carry out specific health activities. In Hong Kong, similarly, many of the mass health campaigns and small capital projects are funded by civic organizations, as well as by professional associations and local government project grants. Communities in Indonesia are granted funds, on presidential instruction, for certain health-related activities, such as the improvement of sanitation and the construction of schools, markets, and health centres. In 11 Indonesian cities assisted by UNICEF, block grants are used for sanitation improvement, income-generating activities, the establishment of a system of community-managed supplementary feeding, etc.

Fig. 9 shows the other types of support required as the community progresses from a state of dependence (A) to the level of self-help (B). In phase 1, support will be required for social analysis, as well as for community organization and the development of

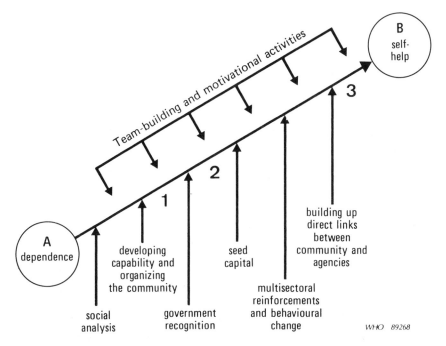

Fig. 9. Organizational and other support for self-help

problem-solving capability. In phase 2, three particular types of support will be needed. Early in this phase, the appropriate community body (e.g., the Health Committee) will need to obtain recognition by the government agency concerned. Then seed capital to initiate projects will be needed. Furthermore, support for activities at the individual, family, and community levels to help sustain a broad range of behavioural changes, leading to better health, will be required. Practical health education can be introduced on such subjects as the proper disposal of garbage, household cleanliness, or personal dental care. Rewards for good performance can be given community-wide publicity.

Finally, in phase 3 (when the community is nearing its self-help level) it is important to provide support for the creation of direct links between the organized community and city agencies. Community leaders must be encouraged to have direct contacts with key staff of the various agencies that are important for the community's activities. The community organizer can facilitate such direct contacts at the outset by bringing agency staff to the community to meet its leaders, and by arranging for the leaders to visit the offices of agencies in the city.

Support for team-building and motivational activities should be provided continuously from the beginning to the end of the process. Other types of support may be needed in all phases, in an *ad hoc* way or at particular times.

Communities and financing

It is a fundamental principle of primary health care that nobody should be denied care on account of poverty. In many of the countries represented at the Manila Consultation (59), though not in all, health care is free for those who cannot afford to pay. Often eligibility is on the basis of some form of assessment of income.

The bulk of the money to pay for health care in poor neighbourhoods must come through reallocation of resources in the health system and elsewhere in public budgets. The cost is modest, the potential impact great, and the case for reallocation overwhelming.

Nevertheless, poor communities should pay something—even if it is only a token amount—for their health care, partly because the contribution of even a modest amount per head helps with the financing, and partly because it is a token of community ownership. The payment need not be in cash. There are, for example, a variety of ways in which community health volunteers can be rewarded or compensated by their neighbours. Equally, community labour can help with sanitation and water supply projects, and even the building of health clinics.

Income-generating schemes (as in Cebu and Manila in the Philippines, or Visakhapatnam in India) also have a very important contribution to make to primary health care and to community development.

Legislation can be used to supplement public money, for example, by requiring local businesses to provide primary health care for their employees, and to contribute to neighbourhood schemes. Local fund-raising (for example, the "United Way" campaign in Baroda, India) and nongovernmental agencies can also help. It is important for communities to participate in the mobilization of funds—apart from what they pay themselves—and in decisions about their use.

In conclusion, there is no doubt today about the importance of community participation in the formulation, design, and delivery of public services, including health care. Resource constraints, as well as the need to choose priorities and to complement what people can do for themselves, would alone require it. Services that people do not want or understand are unlikely to have much impact. But that is actually of secondary significance. What is really important is the principle that all communities, including the poorest, should develop primarily by making choices for themselves, with appropriate advice.

Chapter 4

Health and health-related development in urban areas

Socioeconomic development and health

The link between socioeconomic development and health is a close one. It has been demonstrated by, for example, McKeown in his well known analysis of mortality statistics for England and Wales from the years 1838–41 to the 1970s (76). Similar observations have been made by other people, including the McKinleys, using statistics from the United States (77). McKeown's work helps to clarify, among other things, the probable influences on health status of socioeconomic development and of conventional health service activities, respectively. One result is a strengthening of the case for multisectoral intervention, since so much of what affects health lies outside the scope of medical care, as conventionally defined.

Intersectoral coordination in urban areas

The profound effect on health of income and employment, water supply and sanitation, housing, literacy, and education makes it clear that, although intersectoral coordination often excites more talk than action, it does, in fact, hold the key to any sustained progress.

To be effective, coordination of this sort must operate at several different levels: ministerial, municipal, district, and so on. Quite apart from the government, it is helpful to involve a variety of academic and national institutions, such as institutes of administration, management, public health, or urban affairs, in multidisciplinary baseline studies, surveillance, evaluation, and comparisons between cities. It is also essential, particularly at the local level, to draw upon the efforts of nongovernmental agencies of all kinds, including those in the private sector.

Convergent action by different programmes and sectors entails a considerable effort in terms of intra- and intersectoral linkages.

Action across intersectoral boundaries is seldom easy, and the best means of achieving it is largely open to debate. The point is not so much to contrast and argue over the rival merits of different theoretical models, but to decide for what purposes, or at which stage, a given model is appropriate, and when one should evolve naturally into another. It is primarily a matter of understanding how to mobilize the most appropriate resources to cope with a given problem (irrespective of disciplinary considerations, organizational location, or managerial responsibility) and how to coordinate them all, so that those who can make a useful contribution are involved, gaps are not left, the work is done reasonably efficiently, and the objectives are met. Often there is no perfect way, or perfection would take too long to negotiate. One has to make a start and later adjust the arrangements for intersectoral partnership in the light of experience.

In the urban environment, the health-related problems of water and sanitation, housing, employment, and education absolutely require intersectoral action. The precise mechanisms to be used will, however, depend on the local, district, and city context and, there-fore, no single organizational structure is likely to have wide application. One important point is to identify health-related problems and supply information on their magnitude and causes. This information can then justify the call for support from other sectors and provide a basis for joint action.

Among the points raised at the Manila Consultation (59) on the basis of national experience were:

- Intersectoral collaboration and action must be based on needs identified at the local level, with community involvement.

- Intersectoral collaboration must develop through joint pro-grammes of action, among the agencies that are relevant in the particular case, aimed at solving specific community problems.

- Positive attitudes and commitment on the part of health wor-kers and other personnel involved are crucial; without them, any intersectoral mechanism will be a sham.

- In many countries, the collaboration of nongovernmental or-ganizations needs to be emphasized at both the district level and the policy-making level.

- While the motivation directing health workers to intersectoral collaboration is health, the community itself and the other agencies may have different priorities. This implies a degree of give-and-take, especially if action has to be paid for out of another agency's budget. It also suggests that one should try to economize on the time input required from others. A reliable system of interagency referral may well be more effective than requiring every agency to be represented at every meeting.

- A common problem is a lack of vertical links between coordinating bodies at various levels. Vertical links would be stronger if one representative from each lower-level body was included in the coordinating body at the next higher level.

- Another common problem is lack of good vertical links within the health system, for two-way referral and continued action.

- Links with water, sanitation and other environmental improvement programmes are essential, but often difficult to achieve.

Some examples may be cited. Since 1978, India has gone a long way towards providing basic physical amenities, such as low-cost pour-flush latrines with an on-the-spot disposal system, under environmental improvement schemes in many of its cities. The *Kampung* Improvement Programme in Jakarta, Surabaya, and other Indonesian cities has effectively provided such amenities to nearly all low-income areas. One reason for the programme's effectiveness is that action was taken directly by local authorities and involved specific links with community organizations. In Manila, on the other hand, physical improvements were initiated by the National Housing Authority and appear to have been more limited in coverage and less closely linked to local authorities and community organizations.

While generalizations are dangerous, it appears that cooperative bodies for intersectoral action are likely to work best when the community is the principal partner at the relevant level (neighbourhood, city, etc.) rather than any one agency; when their record is one of tangible achievements; and when they are sparing of people's time. Whatever intersectoral mechanism is evolved for urban primary health care, it is salutary to keep asking *whether it works, why*, and *why not*. Since the need for intersectoral action is inescapable, any coordinating mechanism that does not work has to be made to work or else replaced.

The multiplicity of agencies involved, the many organizational, managerial, financial, and technical problems encountered, and the fact that agencies are primarily answerable to their respective governing bodies—all these make the integration of action difficult from the operational standpoint. Attempts are nevertheless being made to overcome this difficulty. The Delhi Administration, for example, in consultation with the Union Ministry of Health and Family Welfare and the Planning Commission, has defined the roles and responsibilities of individual agencies and is examining a proposal to establish an "apex" health authority (*78*). The Calcutta

114

Metropolitan Development Authority, established as a planning, coordinating, financing and supervising body, has evolved into an effective implementation agency, which has attempted to reverse decades of neglect and to encourage investment outside the "metro-core" (79). It will now revert to its original function. Similar developments have taken place in Bombay and Madras (80). In Mexico City (47), the Secretaría de Salubridad y Asistencia (Health and Welfare Office) coordinates all health care organizations to avoid duplication of services, and real progress has been made in this direction. In Jakarta (47), coordination and guidance to ensure close links between delivery services in low-income urban districts is the responsibility of the Department of Home Affairs. In Kuala Lumpur (81), a special project has been set up by the Ministry of Federal Territory to coordinate the services of agencies within the city that wish to improve the quality of life among the urban poor; it also has direct responsibility for services in the fields of health and family planning, environmental improvement, and community and family development.

Mention should also be made of the Metropolitan Manila Management Conference (82) (January 1981), which discussed and defined priorities, the financing of services, the allocation of resources within the city, and the fostering of interagency relationships in metropolitan management. The Conference proposed the establishment of a form of metropolitan development authority, taking into consideration already existing models. The aim was to achieve a more careful use of resources; greater attention to low-income groups; improved cost recovery, while keeping prices affordable for the poor; and better training in urban management.

Meetings bringing together representatives of several government agencies or ministries can have many positive outcomes, such as improved planning and coordination, innovative ideas, new sources of support, better use of scarce resources, and solutions for problems no agency can solve on its own. Intersectoral collaboration, however, is undeniably difficult and expensive. It is unlikely to be successful unless it focuses on goals of interest to all the parties.

Organizations can be created to promote such collaboration. At country level, for example, a national health council can bring together senior officials for policy decisions, while a national health development network might call upon various institutions and their experts for technical advice on implementation. Regional and district development councils can oversee intersectoral collaboration among representatives of different agencies; intersectoral teams can work on regional problems; and integrated regional projects can provide multiple services. A similar approach can also be taken at city level.

It is also possible to make changes within ministries and municipalities to promote intersectoral collaboration, emphasizing it as a goal valued by leaders. Doing so in a serious way means redefining jobs accordingly, allocating funds for the purpose, and providing incentives for innovative joint ventures with other ministries.

Obtaining adequate support from the higher echelons of the administration is likely to require special efforts to educate senior officials, to increase consultation at all levels and, above all, to establish well-defined policies for decentralization, collaboration, and implementation.

A strategy based on primary health care principles, and clearly articulated, ought to facilitate the allocation of resources, the delegation of authority, and the creation of lines of communication and coordination across sectors, particularly at district and local levels.

The importance of the educational component in preparing for effective intersectoral collaboration can hardly be exaggerated. It must be wide in scope and must operate at various levels, creating awareness at some, changing attitudes at others, and imparting skills in management and coordination to key personnel. In all cases it has to try to overcome resistance to change. Such an extensive programme should include workshops to provide an opportunity for those affected to discuss and understand the changes involved, their likely impact, and the benefits to be expected for each sector. Study tours and secondments to gain practical experience of intersectoral collaboration in other cities, even in other countries, would be useful in obtaining insights into the problems encountered and the ways in which they can be tackled. Visits can also illuminate important sectoral differences in attitudes, values, and expectations.

Intersectoral action should be planned in such a way that the organizational aspects, sectoral roles and responsibilities, and areas and mechanisms of coordination are well defined , together with the parts that nongovernmental agencies are expected to play. Goals should be clearly stated, the anticipated benefits for each sector described, and provision made for the constant monitoring of progress and for regular evaluation by senior management, including politicians.

The plan of action must be developed jointly by all the partners concerned, otherwise there will be serious difficulties sooner or later. Community participation and support, difficult enough to secure at any time, can hardly be expected if essential nongovernmental parties and influential individuals are excluded from the planning phase, and if no real opportunity is provided for them to express their views and describe their needs.

When deciding on the composition and nature of teams for implementation, it is essential to ensure that adequate resources will be available, whether from the central or local government, from other agencies, or through community self-help. Similar provision has to be made for the coordination element of intersectoral action, and this form of recognition should prove a powerful incentive for those concerned. Other types of incentive, including rewards for successful implementation, may also be appropriate. As always, the quality of leadership is of critical importance, and criteria for selection should emphasize goal-orientation and communication skills. For all key posts there should be clear and well-accepted job descriptions, and those occupying them should have a sense of shared strategy.

Lack of community support may be due to a number of factors: apathy, disillusion based on past experience, or simply lack of understanding of the purpose and intended benefits of the particular project or programme. Whatever the causes, a special and sustained effort will be needed to inform the community and to mobilize it into effective participation, whether through committees or through traditional social structures. The matching of grants to stimulate community-initiated intersectoral collaboration can also be helpful.

The approaches outlined apply mainly to the formal aspects of intersectoral collaboration. However, success also depends on the attention paid to more complex and informal processes and relationships, including consultation, cross-sectoral dialogue, informal social contacts, and other forms of "negotiative communication". Those involved in intersectoral collaboration often do not have formal authority over one another and cannot solve problems by issuing direct orders. Negotiation and compromise are thus essential to the achievement of cooperative action.

Intersectoral project for slum improvement in Bangladesh

The urban population of Bangladesh in 1981 was 13 million, approximately 16% of the total population. While there is no official definition of "low income", estimates of the low-income urban population range from 30% to 40% of the urban total, or from 4 to 5 million. The number of urban dwellers is increasing at the rate of 6.5%, more than twice the national growth rate. It is estimated that 70% of the urban growth is due to migration from rural areas.

Data on the health of people in the low-income groups are scarce. It is assumed that their major health problems are similar to those of the country in general, possibly with more malnutrition and diseases related to poor water and sanitation, e.g., diarrhoea.

Government action in the urban areas concentrates on improving water and sanitation. A UNICEF-assisted Slum Improvement Project includes a primary health care component. This pilot project which aims to provide basic services in the cities, started in the town of Mymensingh and will eventually be extended to 16 municipalities. The target population for the project consists of people belonging to households headed by women or households where the women and children earn their living by unskilled labour. They should reside in substandard (*kacha*) housing with household incomes of no more than 800 taka (US$ 27) per month.

The training of community health workers will be a key element in the programme. The health staff of the different municipalities, who at present do very little in the way of providing primary health care, will also be involved. The sanitary inspectors will supervise the community health workers and will receive the same training, plus management training. The district civil surgeons (under the Ministry of Health) will provide technical assistance to the sanitary inspectors. It is hoped that this will encourage closer coordination between the Ministry of Health and the municipalities.

The programme will rely on nongovernmental organizations for assistance in mobilizing communities. However, in urban areas in Bangladesh, very few nongovernmental organizations are working in primary health. The majority of nongovernmental organizations in the cities and towns concentrate on family planning. The exceptions are the Aga Khan Foundation, Project CONCERN (USA), Save the Children (United Kingdom), and Terre des Hommes (Netherlands). Another major group working in urban primary health care consists of volunteers from a research institute dealing with diarrhoeal diseases.

Noakhali became involved in the Slum Improvement Project in the summer of 1986. Previously, no primary health care was available in this city, which has a population of 100 000. Even conventional health services were limited to one government hospital. There were no government health clinics, but two clinics were operated by nongovernmental organizations.

Eventually 2000 families will be involved in the programme. One tube-well for every 10 families and one sanitary latrine for every household will be installed. Some drains, footpaths, and street lights will also be provided through community action, as well as refuse bins and handcarts to carry garbage.

Ten per cent of the cost of the physical improvements will be recovered from (a) the beneficiaries (for tube-wells), (b) the landowners (for sanitary latrines), and (c) the municipalities (for drains, footpaths, street lights, refuse bins). This money will be used to set up a revolving loan fund for slum women.

Women selected by the community to serve as community health workers will be trained locally by a nongovernmental organization. They will be accountable to a "subproject implementation committee" at the slum level.

In each slum, the project will be implemented by groups with specific functions. At the slum level, management will be provided by the subproject implementation committee, composed of the leaders of the different groups. At the municipal level, a project implementation committee will coordinate and manage activities and provide multisectoral support. It will be chaired by the chairman (i.e., the highest elected official) of the municipality, and its members will include public health engineers (water), local government engineers (sanitation, drainage, footpaths), power development officials (street lights), district civil surgeons (health), and others as needed.

Prepared by Mr Fazla Elahi, Chairman Noakhali, Pouzashava, Dhaka, Bangladesh.

Urban development

Good urban development programmes already provide many of the basic ingredients of primary health care, but health authorities often do not take full advantage of the opportunities they offer.

At city level, there are few examples, if any, of a systematic managerial process for tackling the problems of urban deprivation, or of a truly comprehensive city health plan. While there are short- and long-term plans that sometimes reach out to vulnerable groups, they seldom encompass all the relevant needs, resources, and activities. Generally they provide for such conventional measures as creating additional medical facilities, or increasing ratios of health care personnel to population: it is rare for them to give appropriate priority to the things that will actually make the biggest impact on health, such as water supply, sanitation, housing, and nutrition.

There are differences of experience and opinion as regards the desirability of linking health projects closely to large-scale urban development programmes. The problem is that health tends to be relegated to a level of relative insignificance. Nevertheless the urban basic services programme in India and experience in Bogotá provide successful examples of such linkages. Interestingly, the *Kampung* Improvement Programme in Indonesia did not by itself improve health status, despite dramatic improvements in sanitation and water supply. It required a supplementary programme, aimed specifically at promoting healthy behaviour, to reap the health benefits of investment in physical infrastructure.

Of course, some urban development schemes may also have a negative effect on health, if they exacerbate overcrowding, increase immigration, or add to pollution, noise, and other health hazards. All too often, it is the poorest in the community who pay the highest price for such developments (for example, if they live beside high-risk industrial plants) even if others reap a benefit.

Intersectoral coordination and community participation in the Philippines

According to the 1980 census, 45% of the estimated 3.6 million urban households in the Philippines are in the low-income bracket (earning less than 2500 pesos (US$ 120) per month).

A specific framework for the realignment of the health care delivery system in Manila has been adopted. Three major developmental strategies were utilized, namely: strengthening of health services, intersectoral coordination, and research and development.

Health manpower development was given priority through training programmes for health workers of all levels from policy-makers down to those at the grassroots. Management and technical workshops were held to provide the top-level staff with skills in problem-solving and supervision. Various categories of health worker underwent retraining and orientation in primary health care and community development. At the lowest level, *barangay* health volunteers were trained in leadership and health skills. Continuous training—and retraining—is a guiding principle.

Coordination within the health sector between various programmes, with other health agencies, and with government and private hospitals and medical practitioners has been developed to improve health care delivery. A two-way referral system has been established with government hospitals, whereby patients needing only primary medical care are treated at the health centres, while more complicated cases are referred by the health centres to the hospitals.

Much importance is attached to the contributions of various governmental and private agencies to overall community health development, and appropriate intersectoral committees have been created at the city and district levels. The members include agencies concerned with water, housing, food, environmental sanitation, and subsistence, led by the Manila Health Department.

Nongovernmental agencies, social and civic organizations, and religious groups have joined forces with the health centre staff and the community for the implementation of development projects. The Rotary Club of Manila provides financial support for cataract operations, feeding programmes, and "vertical gardens" (a form of backyard vegetable growing). The Union Church of Manila has donated medical equipment and drugs. Small loans are available for income-generating purposes from this religious group, as well as from Business for Social Progress, a civic organization.

A research and development component with a detailed health information system plays a vital part in strengthening the links between the health service system and the community. Experimental communities serve as models and the basis for the expansion of primary health care to other depressed communities in Manila.

Through the *barangay* network and a corps of *barangay* health volunteers, the residents are motivated to get involved in community-based projects and activities. This is an indication of the shift from the traditional paternalistic approach to one of partnership between people and both government and private sectors. One specific project demonstrating self-reliance is the Health Cooperative Scheme and Credit Union. For a fixed monthly contribution, families are assured that essential drugs will be available in case of illness. Small loans may be provided by the Credit Union to enable people to start small businesses to augment family income and help subsidize the insurance scheme.

A very different example comes from Olongapo. Here, in a span of a couple of years, a private teacher-training institution called Columban College was able to give a successful demonstration of an alternative community-based approach to the implementation of primary health care in an urban area. The project was started in 1983, and in 1985 was turned over to the municipality to facilitate the institutionalization of the approach with the local authority's development programme and to prepare for the eventual expansion of the project to other depressed communities.

From the outset, the project team was aware that it could not respond on its own to the problems in the city; that eventually the municipality would have to take over the task of developing, strengthening and expanding basic services in urban low-income communities, with emphasis on strong community organization and community participation.

From the conception of the project to its assessment, every effort was made to ensure that the heads of local government departments were somehow involved, or at least informed. If the project is to be expanded to cover a wider population, it is very important that the local authority should also be socially prepared. Some organizing is therefore necessary at the agency level as well as the community level.

Despite the various problems encountered, or perhaps because of them and the solutions chosen to deal with them, the City Health Officer could not fail to be impressed by the results of the project, particularly the quality of the trained voluntary workers and the community organization's support for community health care.

In the beginning, the City Health Department participated by sharing personnel as motivators and by providing medical supplies and medicine. Soon, it requested UNICEF for assistance in retraining existing community health workers and in training additional ones in the rest of the *barangays*, using Columban College's training curriculum and the services of its staff. When this training had been carried out in all the *barangays* in the city, the parties concerned began to discuss the possibility of expanding the project. Since the City Health Department had the requisite facilities, manpower, and mechanisms for this, it was decided that Columban College should turn the project over to it. It took some breadth of mind on the part of the college to give up the control of the project (but not necessarily its participation in it), and on the part of the City

Health Department to accept the additional responsibilities involved.

In another city in the Philippines, Cebu, the emphasis of the primary health care programme is on income-generating activities. The object is to improve the socioeconomic condition of the people in order to improve their nutritional and health status. As in Manila, the *barangay* health workers play a crucial role. They try to raise funds for the initial outlay, which is often topped up by contributions from nongovernmental organizations. Progress is slow but there are now projects ranging from the sale of barbecued pork, through duck-raising, to shellcraft. The main problem encountered is that the *barangay* health workers find it difficult to remain active in primary health care in view of their own low socioeconomic status and are often obliged to take paid occupations.

Prepared by Dr E. Suva, City Health Officer, Manila Health Department, Dr A. L. Boholst, Medical Supervisor III, Cebu City Health Department, and Mr H. Ruiz, City Health Office, Olongapo City, Philippines.

Employment, income, and nutrition

Unemployment, underemployment, low income, and malnutrition march hand-in-hand with poor health, and attempts to improve the health of the urban poor are not likely to have any lasting effect unless they form part of an overall attack on poverty, involving the creation of jobs and promotion and support for income-generating activities.

Malnutrition is associated with ill health and especially with communicable disease. Not only does it constitute a disease *per se*, but it interacts with other diseases and affects mortality rates (*83*). It has been observed in various cities that, in slums and squatter areas, energy intake is generally one-half to two-thirds the average for the city, vitamin A intake one-third to one-half the average, and anaemia twice as prevalent as it is in the rest of the city. Up to 50% of the children may show signs of malnutrition, 10% of them in a severe form (*41*). Observations from Abidjan (*33*), New Delhi (84, 85), Santiago (*86*), São Paulo (*87*), and various other cities are consistent with these estimates. More important, when the information has been disaggregated by socioeconomic group, it has been found that the availability of nutrients was lower for the urban than for the

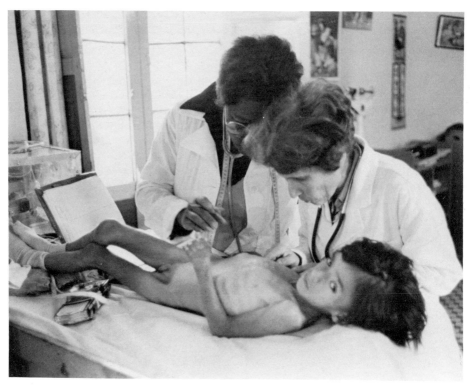

WHO/Y. Pouliquen (17638)

Up to 50% of children in slums and squatter settlements show signs of malnutrition

corresponding rural groups (survey carried out by the National Nutrition Institute in Colombia, 1963–65), or that there were more severely malnourished children in low-income urban areas than in rural areas, as in San José (Costa Rica) (*34*), Guatemala City (*36*), and San Salvador (*35*). It is worth noting that neither the large intra-urban differences observed in the cities of Morocco, nor even the fact that conditions in that country's urban slums are worse than those in its rural areas, would have been apparent if citywide averages had been used in the statistics (*88*).

These findings concerning urban–rural differences are at variance with what is generally believed. Some possible reasons can be mentioned (*89*). Although in South-East Asia and Latin America rural labourers largely depend on their landlords for food, many rural families, especially in Africa, own small pieces of land where they can grow part of their food or avail themselves of harvest surpluses; this is generally not possible for the poor in the over-crowded cities. On the contrary, in the cities, although cash wages

124

are higher, so too are costs, with the result that food itself is more expensive and the poor have a smaller proportion of their income available for it. The observations in Moroccan cities, mentioned above, provide a good example of the fallacy of assuming the same relationship between food availability and income when environmental and social conditions are very different. Furthermore, in the highly competitive conditions of the city, women are often forced to work in full- or part-time jobs (generally in the informal sector) to complement the family income, or as the only family support. Under such circumstances they generally have less time to prepare food. As a result they may resort to early weaning, leave their infants in the care of young children unable to prepare weaning foods properly, have to dilute and eke out a limited milk supply, fall an easy prey to advertising (90), or become victims of various combinations of these possibilities.

Supplementation of family income is directly linked with problems of food and nutrition. Thus, it is an important non-health component of suburban primary health care programmes. The type of income-generating activity employed will vary according to local market conditions and the available materials and skills. Income-generating projects have to be labour-intensive and learning-intensive, if they are to be sustained for any length of time. Otherwise, they will become "hand-outs" and fail in the end. They are most likely to succeed if they are on a small scale, as in the case of cottage industries or one-man businesses, since these are relatively cheap to establish, require little coordination, and yield a direct return to the individuals involved.

It is inadvisable for health staff to serve as direct promoters of income-generating activities without (at the least) careful selection and appropriate training. These are business enterprises, and the knowledge and skills required are totally different from those required for health care.

There are some imaginative and encouraging examples of income-generating activities as part of broad programmes to alleviate poverty, in Bangkok, in Manila and Cebu (Philippines), and in many Indian cities. In Manila, the Health Department has worked closely with the Department of Social Welfare. Training for women and young people has been provided in occupations with a market demand, such as carpentry, dressmaking, and building, the choice being up to the individuals concerned. A range of 21 such activities in Cebu included duck-raising, the making of peanut butter, and the establishment of local general stores (*sari-sari* stores). In Bangkok, income-generating schemes are promoted by the health authorities in collaboration with the Social Welfare Department, on much the same lines as in Manila. Sometimes income-generating activities form a natural adjunct to other health care activities, for example, growing herbs, preparing herbal remedies, and packaging or retailing healthy foods.

Also in Manila, civic groups and other government agencies were persuaded to lend families the capital for such undertakings as paper-bag manufacture, *sari-sari* stores, and "rolling" stores (selling goods to motorists and passengers temporarily held up in traffic jams).

Low-income housing

In a recent review, Yeh (*91*) describes experience in 6 cities (Bangkok, Hong Kong, Jakarta, Kuala Lumpur, Manila, and Singapore) and draws the conclusion that it is unrealistic for the large countries of South-East Asia to expect to solve their housing problems in the present decade, given the rate of urban population growth and the rapid increase in slum and squatter areas.

Many so-called low-income housing projects have resulted in the displacement of the urban poor and their replacement by relatively well-off families. Thus, the poor remain badly housed and may even become poorer. It is essential to reduce requirements for housing standards to realistic levels and to provide affordable housing units that can be gradually improved. In Nairobi, for example, a nongovernmental organization helped slum dwellers to build their own houses at a fraction of the cost of a major governmental and international scheme nearby. Leaving aside the obvious advantages of lower costs, there is no proof that, once certain minimum requirements are fulfilled (*92*), more expensive housing will necessarily produce better health.

Hong Kong and Singapore are special cases, but have met 50% and 75%, respectively, of their requirements with public housing, its provision at affordable cost being only part of an overall programme of social development, which includes education, health, and the expansion of employment. It seems probable that the secret of their success lies in their comprehensive approach and the changes in political thinking, legislation, administration, and resource allocation that this has entailed. Without such an approach it is unlikely that other cities can make significant progress in this field.

Well-planned, low-cost housing schemes improve the health of the community, not so much because of better accommodation but because of the amenities and facilities that go with them—water

126

supply, sanitation, access to employment, and education. Money can be raised from officially sponsored low-cost housing schemes to pay for health care, through small additions to rents or loan repayments, even when direct charges for health care are not judged acceptable.

In the past, some ill-conceived slum upgrading and slum clearance programmes have left the poor in a worse state than before. Forced movement to a different site means social disruption, and often greater distances from work and higher transport costs. High rent, even for much better housing, means less money for food.

That is not to deny the contribution that housing can make, since shelter, clean water, and sanitation are fundamental to health. But it is an argument for simple, inexpensive solutions in housing, as in primary health care. The link between the two is very clear. A good example is the Million Houses Programme in Sri Lanka, the chairman of which is the coordinator at national level of the Urban Basic Services Programme, based on the primary health care approach. Another example is Maputo City (Mozambique), which is organizing the urbanization of new neighbourhoods where people with the lowest incomes can build their own homes. Because water supply and low-cost sanitation are an integral part of this programme, these new neighbourhoods are actually healthier than many older ones, even though the people in the latter may have higher incomes.

The process of improving environmental health conditions requires guidelines and methods that can be adapted and used. A recent WHO publication (*93*) recommended methods for the promotional, survey, planning, implementation, monitoring, and evaluation phases of this process.

Legislation and legalization

Appropriate legislation promotes and protects the health of the population. However, the enforcement of outdated laws and standards that are no longer appropriate can only limit progress or have a deleterious effect on the health of a community. Thus, adherence to zoning laws and building standards adopted many years ago may exclude the poor from living near the industrial, commercial, or high-income residential areas where work may be found. Similarly, building codes designed for a more affluent age put legally acceptable construction beyond the reach of the poorer sections of the population. Such laws and regulations need to be revised to respond to today's realities.

Legalization of tenure is a fundamental issue for the millions who live in squatters' settlements. Without legal status, these people, already among the poorest, may often be denied the social benefits to which they might otherwise be entitled. Moreover, it is obvious, in cities such as Guayaquil or Manila, that dramatic improvements often begin the moment people achieve some security of tenure. India, the Philippines, and Thailand provide relevant examples of urban land reform. In India, for example, state governments have passed slum improvement acts under which land is acquired for the poor with government funds, and title deeds are then distributed free.

It is not difficult to see that, where migration into the cities is continuing, landlords and enforcers of regulations are constantly faced with unmanageable problems. People may well settle in places where they are in real physical danger (from high-tension wires, for example, or in flood zones) or where they create a nuisance. There are no easy answers to these problems. But measures to allow those in desperate need to find shelter must be an essential priority. To the extent that the enforcement of rules, zoning regulations, etc. is necessary, communities in poor neighbourhoods may themselves be the most effective enforcers, if they understand why the rules are required. At all events, regulations will continually be flouted in most countries, if enforcement depends solely on external force.

Another need is for legal aid (provided, for example, in India under a special budget) to assist the urban poor in defending themselves and upholding their legal rights as citizens. The poor often become vicitims of law enforcement agencies, without adequate defence even when their case is good.

Water supply and sanitation

Nobody should underestimate the influence of water supply and sanitation on health. Arguably they are, along with nutrition, the most important factors involved, having a greater impact than any activity of the health services proper.

The lack of safe water and of appropriate sanitation is one of the leading causes of morbidity and mortality in developing countries, contributing every year to some 4–5 million deaths of infants and young children from diarrhoea (94).

The following table summarizes the changes in coverage by urban water supply and sanitation services between 1975 and 1985 (95).

	Year		
	1975	*1980*	*1985*
Urban water supply			
no. of countries reporting	76	81	89
total population (millions)	502	593	727
coverage (millions/percentage of total population)	372/74	431/73	543/75
Urban sanitation			
no. of countries reporting	60	78	77
total population (millions)	376	591	683
coverage (millions/percentage of total population)	192/51	292/49	401/59

While these figures show some improvements in coverage, they also show that large numbers of people remain unserved. In most cases these are the poorest, and therefore most vulnerable, sections of the urban communities concerned.

In Juba (Sudan), for example, there was a cholera outbreak in 1979. It was mainly the poor who were affected, because they took their drinking-water from a contaminated river. Bore-wells were sunk after that, but were not maintained, because people objected to the high salt content of the water and started using the river again, not recognizing the risks. Water tankers were developed as yet another solution, which seems to be working, but at the high price of 1.25 Sudanese pounds per drum.

In view of the scale of the problems that are still outstanding in the areas of water supply and sanitation, and the lack of resources to pay for conventional capital-intensive schemes, emphasis has to be placed (as with housing) on low-cost, appropriate options and community participation. Fortunately, encouraging examples exist in Bangkok, Colombo, Karachi, and elsewhere. In Colombo, a slum population of 40 000 installed community latrines (one for every 5 families) over a period of two years.

In Karachi, in the Orangi project, a school of architecture, a nongovernmental organization, and local communities collaborated to produce (through free local labour) an effective low-cost water supply and sewerage system. The communities participated in the planning, and the architectural students did the technical designs as part of their course. In India, a voluntary organization called Sulabh International has built several public latrines in collaboration with the municipal authority concerned and maintains them on a "pay-for-use" principle.

In rural areas the need for water supplies is greater than the need for improved sanitation: in urban areas, because of lack of space and high population densities, both are fundamentally important. However, governments and landlords are often reluctant to invest in areas that they consider to be illegally occupied and that are likely to be cleared. The situation is aggravated by the tendency to consider only high-cost conventional solutions to the problems of the slums, and to reject alternative, decentralized methods that cost less but that may be effective, provided that they have the support of the residents and the physical measures applied are accompanied by behavioural changes.

The people themselves may exacerbate the problem. Their view of priorities is naturally influenced by the immediacy of their needs and the visibility of the results. For a mother with a sick child, for example, medical treatment and the money to pay for it are what really counts at that moment. Or people may be unconcerned with the need for regular maintenance and adopt the attitude that "it's the government's job to collect the garbage" (96). Worse, they may make illegal water connections and, in doing so, contribute to the deterioration of the supply, complete with leakage, waste, and contamination. These problems can be dealt with only by adopting an approach based on community participation.

Population density is obviously relevant, not only in terms of numbers of people to be served, but because it influences the choice of systems. Densities are often extremely high: in the old city of Kabul in 1975, the housing situation of 37% of the 541 000 inhabitants was such that more than two families had to live in one unit, and two or three persons in one room. In Old Delhi there are as many as 270 000 people per km² (97). In the *medina* of Casablanca the average density is 70 000 per km² (10 times more than in the city's well-to-do residential areas). In the three towns of Ghana that have more than 50 000 people, 35% of the population live at least 20 to a house. Three-quarters of Bombay's families live in one room or share a room with another family (98). This type of situation clearly demands that more attention be paid to the adequate provision of water and sanitation.

The availability of a piped system for drinking-water does not by itself ensure the supply expected: relative scarcity of water in relation to the numbers to be served, low pressure, and intermittent delivery may make for a very unsatisfactory service. Several sources of supply are generally available. For example, a report published in 1972 (99) stated that, in the Klong Toey settlement of Bangkok, which had a population of 30 000, 55% of the dwelling units depended on water purchased from vendors; 30% of them were

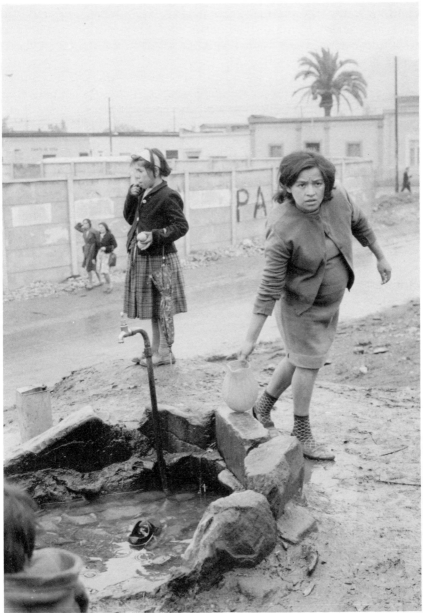

WHO/P. Almasy (12062)

A safe water supply is a prerequisite for good health

served by running water supplied from the city main to a neighbouring house; 3% by house connections to the city main; 10% by running water from a nearby tap; and 1% by rainwater. In a Seoul squatter settlement, water may be available from public taps only in the middle of the night, when demand is low in the more privileged sections of the city (*100*).

Likewise, a variety of means are used to dispose of human wastes. The most common are: defecation trenches (not practical in most cities owing to limited space); "wrap and carry" (where there are places for dumping close by); bucket and overhung latrines above tidal flats, weirs, canals, or beaches (but serious problems arise where water is stagnant or is used for domestic purposes); and wet and dry pit-latrines (quite common but difficult to maintain and highly contaminating).

Equally inadequate are the methods of garbage disposal. To qualify theoretically for having one's refuse collected by the municipal service, as in long-established slums, does not guarantee its removal: in that case, the alternative is to dump it in the street. Many squatter settlements are built near, or on, garbage dumps. In several cities a large informal industry has developed, known in Japanese as the "regenerated resources industry", which consists of gleaning, dealing in, and processing the contents of the dumps. Children are often the ones who pick over the garbage. The health risks involved in this activity are obvious.

Governments and international organizations taking part in the improvement of water supply and sanitation systems have usually given priority to rural projects, because the majority of people in most developing countries still live in rural areas and because this may help to slow down rural–urban migration. However, it is now evident that the situation of those living in slums and shanty towns calls for urgent attention. Here, epidemiological and technical, as well as humanitarian, considerations point to the provision of water and sanitation as not only the single most important line of action, but one that will give lasting results. Measures in respect of land ownership, as well as better housing and attacks on specific diseases (e.g., synchronized deworming and vector control), could extend and consolidate the benefits. One-third of the 1979 investment of the World Bank in water and sanitation was devoted to relieving urban poverty, using the "site-and-service" or "slum-upgrading" approaches. Unfortunately, new investments of this kind often cannot keep pace with a rapidly deteriorating situation; and sometimes speculation and manipulation may prevent the intended beneficiaries from actually benefiting (*101*).

With an anticipated urban population of some 2000 million in the developing regions of the world by the year 2000, it is clear that the International Drinking Water Supply and Sanitation Decade's target of world coverage by 1990 will not be achieved. Moreover, as the term "sanitation" is generally not taken to include disposal of solid wastes and sullage, as far as the Decade is concerned, a net deterioration in sanitation is a possibility.

The developing world is littered with broken-down or badly functioning water and sanitation facilities (*102*). Quite apart from the wasted investment they represent and their danger to the population, these defective systems traditionally have had a strong demotivating effect and discourage future investment. However, the reorientation of projects to incorporate the community partnership approach is now gaining momentum.

The rehabilitation of water supply systems is an urgent need. In the Americas, for example, it has been estimated that control of leaks alone could provide enough extra water to meet the additional needs created by the growth in population expected during the Decade.

In most cases, new investment to provide substitute services turns out to be considerably more expensive than rehabilitation, and the problem of poor operation and maintenance remains unresolved. Rehabilitation is now generally recognized as the first option to be considered. Yet new construction is still often favoured, both in development plans and, in many cases, by financing institutions or bilateral aid agencies.

The recommended emphasis on rehabilitation and on correcting operational and maintenance deficiencies implies a change of direction, not only by water agencies and government departments in the developing countries but, equally, by those providing outside support, either financial or technical. In this context, the International Drinking Water Supply and Sanitation Decade advocates the following policy: "In urban areas, developing countries, with the aid of external support agencies where required, should establish a *cost-recovery strategy* based on the criteria of: making drinking water and sanitation accessible to all segments of the population; ensuring the gradual financial autonomy of the water supply and sanitation agency; and discouraging the waste of water. Full cost recovery (operation and maintenance, depreciation of equipment, and debt servicing) is a long-term objective, to be reached preferably by cross-subsidizing tariffs. No single group of the population should be privileged by external subsidies (e.g. for household or yard connections) while other groups in the project area have no access to any reliable water supply" (*103*).

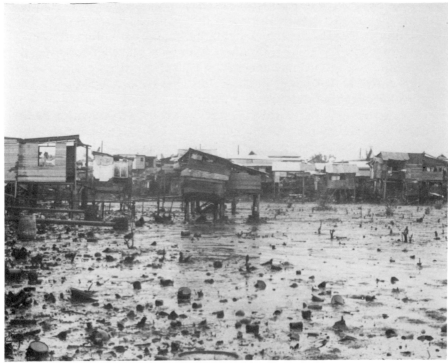

WHO (329)

The appalling litter and decay of a community for which nobody cares

Literacy and education

Education is decisive in improving health and reducing mortality; this applies especially to a number of the developing countries (*104*). Even a few years of schooling make a vital difference to the individual's capacity to handle situations. Poor countries that have given priority to investment in education have reduced their mortality rates far below those of countries with much higher per capita incomes but less educated populations.

Wide differentials in child survival are closely related to the differences in the educational level of the mothers. Child mortality declines as maternal education increases. Even in towns with adequate health facilities, infant mortality rates remain high in families where the mother is illiterate. There is also a close correlation between the educational level of women and their acceptance of family planning.

134

Where the level of female literacy is low, educational strategy should give priority to achieving universal primary education. At the same time, the existing problem of illiteracy among adult females has to be dealt with by imparting functional literacy and by non-formal education, including knowledge about health.

Action by women constitutes one of the most vital forces for health around the world. In China, for example, the Women's Federation oversees day-care centres and literacy campaigns, and makes monthly visits to young children. While Chinese women do this as a regular, understood duty, there is nevertheless an urgent need to improve their managerial skills at different levels so that their action may be even more effective.

The education of women in low-income groups helps them to understand the benefits of breast-feeding, of a balanced uncontaminated diet for their children, and of personal hygiene. It is associated with lower fertility levels (*105*) and increases the efficiency of family planning programmes. Of particular value also is the concept of "basic education" (*106*) which differs from conventional primary education in the sense that it attempts to satisfy the minimum needs of specifically identified groups—not only children but also young people, men and women, and selected rural and urban groups.

School feeding programmes are not only an incentive to the enrolment of children in schools but also a means to better health, regular attendance, and the ability and motivation to learn (*107*).

Teachers and schools can play a very useful role in health. The "little doctor" programme in Indonesia effectively mobilizes the nation's children to understand their own health and to influence their parents. Several cities around the world have school-based health programmes. Seventh- and eighth-grade Colombian students, in preparation for their work in the ninth grade, receive practical training in maternal and child health in two or three families each.

Schools and schoolteachers thus represent a potential health resource, the value of which is often not realized and remains unexplored. Schools are a meeting-place for the community, the teachers are better educated than the majority of the local population, and schoolchildren (and, through them, their parents) are a captive audience in the most receptive and impressionable years of their lives. The years spent in school can do much to determine the future health of the community. The closest collaboration should therefore be maintained between health and education authorities and workers, from the governmental and administrative levels right down to the neighbourhood schools.

To plan a community health programme without involving schools and their teachers is to invite failure. With a little training, teachers can monitor the health of the children in their charge, refer them to the health centre when necessary, supervise feeding programmes, assist in immunization programmes, treat trachoma and iron-deficiency anaemia, take part in programmes for helminthiasis control, and ensure that health promotion and disease prevention are well and imaginatively taught in the schools.

An important step is for health authorities to help the Ministry of Education to introduce an appropriate health education component at all stages of primary and secondary education, and to ensure that teachers receive a thorough preparation for work in this area at their training colleges.

The situation in Addis Ababa

Urban primary health care in Ethiopia follows national policy in this field. Individuals with a monthly income of less than US$ 25 per month are eligible for free health care. Separate health data are not available for low-income urban populations, but in urban areas as a whole 27–40% of children weigh less than 80% of the Harvard standard weight-for-age.

Addis Ababa, a city with 1.5 million people, is socially and politically organized into 284 *kebeles* (urban dwellers' associations) grouped so as to form 25 "higher" *kebeles*.

On the basis of this infrastructure, urban primary health care was launched in 1984. The training of community health agents for 3 months was conducted at the Addis Ababa regional health department. To assist these agents in data collection and other activities, another group of volunteers called "animators" was also trained. There are 276 of the former, and 1139 of the latter. In addition, there are also 153 traditional birth attendants. Only the community health agents are paid; as municipal employees, they have other duties and responsibilities. In every *kebele* (usually about 3000–4000 people), there is a health committee which facilitates coordination between sectors. Current emphasis in the programme is on immunization and health education.

The primary health care programme in Addis Ababa is a good example of different institutions working together—in this case the Ministry of Health (which covers all health institutions), the municipality (which is responsible for the *kebeles*), and UNICEF (which provides material and financial support).

The local nongovernmental organizations in the city have shown a great deal of initiative in establishing health programmes in certain *kebeles*. These include the provision of safe water supplies, the establishment of kitchen gardens, and the development of income-generating schemes.

Community involvement in all these undertakings is facilitated by the existing political structure of the *kebeles*, which include youth and women's associations.

Perceived obstacles to the progress of urban primary health care are: shortage of safe water; poor housing; shortage of funds; insufficient support for community health workers; and poor supervision of community health workers.

Prepared by Mr Duguma Alenayhu, Regional Community Health Agent Coordinator, Addis Ababa, and Mr H. Wubneh, Primary Health Care Coordinator, Ministry of Health, Addis Ababa, Ethiopia.

Multisectoral projects with a health component

The appeal and feasibility of the multisectoral approach, and the confidence that it commands at the community level, are demonstrated by the number, variety, and continuing proliferation of projects employing it. In both rural and urban districts, an attempt must be made to look at health problems without the distorting effect of disciplinary or sectoral considerations, on the basis of their true determinants, their relative importance, and their chronological relationship. Indeed it was from relatively recent initiatives along these lines that the primary health care concept and strategy evolved.

In the case of urban populations in general and of the urban poor in particular, social, environmental, and economic conditions, individual and community behaviour, health status, and general well-being are so closely and intricately linked that no lasting solution to the prevailing problems can be envisaged that does not give due weight to all the relevant elements in proportion to their importance.

On the basis of surveys carried out in 1977 in Addis Ababa, in which the local university took part, an urban upgrading programme was initiated, the main emphasis being on mothers and children in the most deprived *kebeles*. Forty per cent of the urban population of Ethiopia lives in Addis Ababa, and 80–90% of the city's population is below the poverty line, living in crowded low-grade settlements without essential services. The programme includes supplementary feeding, promotion of child and day-care centres, training of day-care instructors, development of small-scale poultry farming and market-gardening, and integrated slum rehabilitation. Several national and international organizations have taken part, their activities being coordinated by the Ministry of Labour and Social Affairs. Women's organizations play a fundamental role. Progress is being made in spite of such constraints as a shortage of manpower, equipment, educational material, and finance, and a steep rise in prices after 1978.

Hyderabad, one of 14 cities in which the Indian Government has undertaken experimental urban community projects after deciding in 1966 to shift from "slum eradication" to "slum improvement" (*108*), has experienced a rapid increase in population. It is now the fifth largest city in India with an estimated 2.5 million inhabitants, of whom 500 000 live in slums. The project is comprehensive and includes: environmental sanitation, the construction of "self-help" houses and of an improved water supply system, family welfare, immunization, health and first-aid classes, family planning, cooking and home-marketing demonstrations, supplementary feeding, special nutrition and midday-meal programmes, recreational and cultural activities and youth programmes, crèches, primary and night schools, vocational training, and economic support through bank loans and activities such as sewing cooperatives. Special emphasis is placed on the participation of women, on ways in which they can supplement the family income, and on their inclusion in the project staff. In spite of the usual problems regarding management and the scarcity of manpower, the project is expanding and is being replicated in other States.

The Sang Kancil[1] project was started in 1979 in Kuala Lumpur to meet the numerous health problems of the large squatter population, which had risen dramatically during the previous 10 years (*109, 110*). A 1978 census of the squatters recorded 48 709 households distributed among 148 squatter settlements and containing a population of at least 234 000, out of a total of about one million for the city as a whole. A consultative seminar in 1978 concluded that there was a high risk of communicable diseases in the squatter communities, where less than 30% of the children had been immunized and there was a high prevalence of worm infestations; that the care of poor children should be closely linked to that of their mothers; that emotional problems, truancy, and drug addiction were

---

[1] Named after the clever mouse-deer (chevrotain), which is a character in popular children's stories in Malaysia.

extremely frequent among schoolchildren; and that a high proportion of working mothers had to leave their children with neighbours, with other children, or on their own. After extensive consultation, the Sang Kancil project opted to focus on preschool education, maternal and child care, and income-generating activities. Community centres were constructed in two areas with the intention of having 20 such centres by 1985. Two kinds of personnel have been trained: the nurse-practitioner, and the community preschool teacher. Income-generating activities were the most difficult to develop, but were considered a very important component of the project, because of the relationship between income and health. A first step was the establishment of a "mini-factory" where women from squatter settlements learned needlecraft, tailoring, and the manufacture of batik garments and soft toys, thus being able to increase their income by 25%.

A project in the poor areas (called "young towns") of the southern zone of Metropolitan Lima was initiated in 1978 to cover 45 neighbourhoods with a total population of about 550 000 (*111*). Its objective is integrated health care for the child and the family at the primary level, through coordinated action by services, institutions, and organized communities. The conditions in which the people of the "young towns" live are harsh, being characterized by underemployment, malnutrition, occupational difficulties, little access to basic services, and so on. Fifty-four per cent of the population have no stable employment, and almost 60% are unable to obtain more than 80% of their caloric needs. Infant mortality is high, and medical services are inadequate. Almost 6000 tons of garbage are dumped each month on the periphery of the settlements. Only 7% of the population have a domestic piped-water supply and sewerage services. The situation of the women is particularly bad, largely because of the traditional attitude that they should not study or work outside the home. Because of the size of the settlements and the high proportion of the total metropolitan population living there, these socioeconomic and physical conditions represent a major policy issue for the country and government. The project activities comprise: mother and child care, including nutrition and oral health; water supply and environmental sanitation; early mental stimulation and non-formal initial education of children; basic education and training of women in dressmaking, shoemaking, food processing, carpentry, and other skills; and the training of block monitors, health promoters, and midwives. The project is based on a thorough analysis of conditions and relies on local community organizations. Initially it covered 46 "young towns", and it is being expanded to other areas.

Rocinha, one of the largest, but not one of the worst, *favelas* of Rio de Janeiro, is rather heterogeneous, with some semi-legalized areas and, especially on the steep slopes, areas where the population lives under very precarious conditions of extreme indigence (*71*). The most striking feature is the accumulation of human wastes and garbage, with all the likely consequences in terms of disease, and insect and rodent infestation. There is a history of community organization, some local services being supported by community groups. The components of the programme include water supply and sanitation, informal education, community schools, day care, and primary health care. Progress is being made in all of them. A notable degree of community participation has been achieved, and the programme has demonstrated that community resources and public support can produce favourable results. The work is being extended to other *favelas*, using the methodology developed in Rocinha.

Other examples are available from the Mathare Valley (Kenya), Rosso (Mauritania), Maxquene (Mozambique), and various districts in Dakar, Dar-es-Salaam, and elsewhere.

Projects of the type described play an important part in changing attitudes and priorities, provided that a number of specific requirements are met. Thus, they must be planned with a long-term perspective (e.g., a 10-year horizon). There has to be considerable initial investment of staff, time, and skills to bring them to the point of take-off. There must also be real involvement of the communities served, which must understand and support the project. Political leaders must be able to assess for themselves the nature and impact of the projects. Finally, the introduction of primary health care through such projects should, from the beginning, be regarded as the first step in a strategy for large-scale action to extend health care to all those previously neglected in this respect.

Chapter 5

Towards universal coverage

Health for all: responsibility of all

Health as a shared responsibility of all individuals, communities, sectors, and organizations is one of the most innovative concepts of the World Health Organization's health for all strategy. In slums and shanty towns, the extremely poor social and environmental conditions and the unhealthy behaviour of the people have a dominant and destructive influence on health. Improvement calls for the combined efforts of a variety of government agencies, and community action has an important part to play. Much remains to be done to remove the constraining effects of sectoral boundaries and bureaucratic compartmentalization, and to develop and implement properly targeted multisectoral action. But encouraging initiatives already exist, and there is no reason to think that such initiatives will not become more common in the future. For example, with the support of organizations like the World Bank, a substantial investment of national and international resources has already been made in multisectoral projects to improve environmental conditions in slums and shanty towns. Even if health is not an explicit goal in many of these projects, they will have favourable effects on health. In fact, some of them offer scope for the incorporation of a health component or for monitoring effects on health. In other cities various health programmes have been established on the initiative of the community, with government agencies and other organizations becoming partners, rather than the other way round. Most of these programmes are based on a multisectoral pattern of interventions. All this indicates that community involvement is useful and, on a long-term basis, may be the only viable approach. Likewise, intersectoral coordination, which is often so difficult and ineffective at higher levels, is natural and realistic at the community level.

The primary health care approach to health for all has been endorsed at the international level by practically all the countries of the world. The strategy requires priority action in favour of deprived populations, be they rural or urban. At country level, however, its translation into concrete action is conditioned by national realities. Understanding of the concepts on which the Declaration of Alma-Ata is based is not widespread, even among members of the health care professions. Despite all the efforts made, the reorientation of national health systems and the redistribution of resources in line with these concepts are still far from being achieved (*112*). An enormous effort is still required to educate the public and to train medical and other health personnel.

In most cities, health facilities and services are inequitably distributed, oriented primarily to dealing with established disease rather than prevention, too expensive and, perhaps, unnecessarily sophisticated. There are nevertheless some notable examples of cities where action has been taken to increase the utilization of peripheral health units, redistribute the patient workload within the city more efficiently, and improve referral. Through various forms of health education and an intelligent use of mass media, awareness of disease causation has been improved, self-help has been stimulated, and healthy behaviour promoted. The reactionary attitude of traditional health services is being changed through the promotion of neighbourhood health teams and programmes, and the training and deployment of an increasing number of community health workers. The big challenges remain the same: the integration of the various initiatives cited, their expansion to achieve total coverage, and the maintenance of the effort required to sustain them in the long term.

National strategies for urban health systems

As a UNICEF/WHO meeting held in July 1983 concluded (*47*): "the plight of those living in the slums and shanty towns of the developing world is one of the most important, yet least understood, problems facing the human race. Many worthwhile projects are now in place, and there is an increasing fund of experience on which to draw. More people need to be aware of the scale and urgency of the problem, and of the approaches that should prove relevant, particularly those in positions of leadership in the cities and countries of the developing world and in international organizations. Above all, more action is needed and rapid scaling-up of current efforts from isolated initiatives, until primary health care for people at risk in urban areas becomes a central component of national and international health care strategies."

A framework for national health care strategies has been formulated in the "Declaration on Strengthening District Health

Systems Based on Primary Health Care" made in Harare, Zimbabwe, on 7 August 1987 (*113*).

Even though many cities are largely autonomous in the conduct of their health services, their policies should be developed within an overall national strategy for urban health in general, and primary health care in particular. The essential target of this strategy should be the universal coverage of urban districts by primary health care. Such a policy should, of course, be matched by a comparable policy for rural areas, though the speed and manner of implementation would necessarily be different.

There are some instances of the formulation of an urban policy giving priority to the problems of slums and shanty towns, followed by the drafting of appropriate plans and programmes. These, however, are still few and far between. And even where such plans and programmes do exist, their implementation has encountered all sorts of barriers. Additional resources have been hard to come by in times of oil crises and economic recession. It follows that little can be done without a redistribution of resources within the urban health system. Indeed, such a redistribution is the most fundamental indication that things are really changing. Yet it has rarely materialized, because of the imperatives of existing commitments, the resistance of conservative groups, or just people's sheer ignorance of the situation.

Government initiatives to improve the level of health in urban districts should concentrate on the slums and shanty towns, emphasizing the upgrading rather than the clearance of slum and squatter areas. If additional resources become available they should be allocated preferentially to meeting the needs of deprived groups. If no additional resources can be obtained, a reallocation of what is already available within the urban health system will have to be undertaken, in order to achieve a more equitable and more effective distribution of services among various districts and communities.

Strengthening ministries of health for primary health care

What does the strengthening of ministries of health for primary health care mean? At first glance, "strengthening" might mean upgrading the qualifications of health workers, expanding health budgets, improving quality control, and ensuring that ministries have a powerful voice in national policy-making. Thus, a stronger ministry would be one with more highly trained staff, greater financial resources, better control of health services, and the ability to influence policy in other ministries and local government bodies to fit health priorities.

But, if the ultimate purpose is to strengthen primary health care, then the definitions suggested above may be wrong. Ministries are only strong if they are able to use all the available resources to provide better and more equitable health care. They are not "strong" if they train more highly qualified doctors at the expense of training auxiliaries and community health workers; if they invest scarce funds in sophisticated tertiary hospitals when the needs of health centres and mobile services within some districts of the city are still unmet; if they use highly qualified staff for simple health measures that might be undertaken by others; if they direct national policies towards narrow health concerns instead of major developmental needs. In short, whether health ministries are "strong" must be judged in the context of primary health care objectives.

The subject was recently considered by a WHO Expert Committee (*114*), which reviewed the functions of ministries of health in the context of the national health system infrastructure and, having identified their weaknesses, recommended seven strategies to strengthen them for primary health care, as follows:

— determination of the appropriate scope of ministry of health responsibilities;

— coordination of functions within the health sector;

— decentralization and organizational restructuring;

— improvement of management and leadership;

— intersectoral collaboration;

— community involvement; and

— increased economic support.

These strategies are all relevant to, and important for, the implementation of primary health care, whether urban or rural, and apply as much to a municipal health department as to a ministry of health, though in different degrees.

Furthermore, they all require examination and appropriate action before any significant expansion of primary health care programmes to achieve wider coverage can be undertaken.

From projects to major programmes

"Scaling-up" (or the implementation of a project on a uniform national basis) is a perennial problem in development. The last three decades have been mainly characterized by limited or pilot projects which, though good, lead others nowhere. They are like islands in a sea of inertia.

Nor is expansion from projects to more broadly based programmes the only problem. In some countries (Colombia, for example) there are programmes of primary health care dating back a quarter of a century, i.e., to long before the Declaration of Alma-Ata, which must be reckoned successes by most standards—except for their lack of impact on the rest of the health care system. Despite their example, there still remain large groups of people—particularly poor people—not covered by basic health care. As yet, the health system as a whole shows little sign of making the fundamental adjustments required. For no health system can be effective that lacks a comprehensive, low-cost service of first contact or fails to use its more sophisticated and expensive resources in support of a primary health care network.

Success on a small scale, particularly in the early days of a project or programme, often depends on a few enthusiastic, highly motivated, and charismatic individuals: these are exceptional people.

Achieving major changes in a large public service demands skill in the management of big bureaucratic organizations, political astuteness, and sheer dogged persistence. Often there is inadequate logistic support and too few trained staff to move from small-scale to large-scale success. At times, too, the planners and policy-makers are sceptical or defeatist. They do not believe the objective can be achieved in the foreseeable future, so very little happens.

Replicating a successful local model nationally is likely to pose at least two problems. On the one hand no single model, however good, will fit all circumstances in every region. On the other hand, it may well not be feasible—in the short term at least—to devise a programme that is tailored to the specific circumstances of each locality. Yet there may be strong political pressure to allocate evenly whatever resources can be made available for primary health care, rather than concentrate them in particular areas sequentially.

Ultimately, expansion is a political decision which should establish priorities, channel the necessary resources, and establish a political and management process to develop an appropriate plan of action.

Such a plan should take account of two important elements:

1. the need to choose priorities in terms of:
   — population groups, concentrating on those in greatest need;
   — geographical areas (because of their variety and the impossibility of doing everything at once);

—measures that will have an impact and a good chance of success;

2. the need to establish concrete objectives for the short, medium, and long term that can be reached through phases of expansion and are realistically linked to the resources available. The criteria for the measures that should have priority are, basically, effectiveness and feasibility.

A number of important constraints stand in the way of implementation of primary health care:

● *The inputs of financial and human resources in pilot projects are often too great to be widely replicable within existing resources.* These inputs include finance, technical assistance, staff, volunteers, supplies, equipment, and infrastructural support from government bodies, voluntary organizations, and international development agencies. The lower the cost and the lower the number of outside inputs, the more possibility there is of replication and of extending the lessons learnt to the health care system as a whole.

● *Any single "standard package" may not have enough flexibility to be adapted to a wide variety of local situations and cultural contexts.* How can a large-scale government programme be flexibly implemented? What are the constraints? What positive factors help? Can the approach be flexible enough to take up issues outside the health sector? The more flexible the approach, the more likelihood there is of its finding acceptance locally. Greater decentralization may help towards achieving such flexibility.

● *Often voluntary organizations have initiated projects with little or no involvement of government; thus they have failed to take the real-life constraints of government bureaucracy into account and the projects lack credibility.* The closer the contact with the government, the more credible the project and the greater the possibility of its being replicated. On the other hand, voluntary organizations are sometimes rightfully distrustful of the stultifying effect of early government intervention.

● *Sometimes there is not enough community involvement at all the stages of a project to ensure appropriateness, cost-effectiveness, coverage, and continuity.* The more the community is involved, the greater the possibility of adaptation, extension, and continuity.

146

- *Sometimes the initiators of a programme try to expand it and establish it on a national scale too quickly.* An over-hasty approach may not leave enough time to explain the programme and to prepare and train people for it. A long-term view is necessary. Expansion, in terms of both geography and range of activities, should be a gradual, phased process. One must avoid trying to do everything, everywhere, at once.

- *The attitudes of government officials and professionals are sometimes major constraints.* Those in authority often do not trust people enough or believe they have the capacity to take responsibility for their own health and well-being. On the contrary, everyone has a brain and can use it in what he/she judges to be his/her own best interests. People are likely to be more often right than wrong in such judgements.

- *Officials are also often sceptical or suspicious of voluntary agencies,* failing to recognize their great potential as instruments of development.

- *Doctors and other professional health care workers may be suspicious of, and resistant to, such a radically new approach.* In this case, they have to be prepared and involved, just as do the urban poor. The more cooperation there is from the people, the voluntary organizations, and the medical profession, the greater the possibility of scaling up activities and changing the broader system of health care.

Scaling-up will be easier if demonstration projects take account from the beginning of the need for their subsequent extension and replicability. It will also be helpful if they can be added to in a modular way, to cover additional neighbourhoods and to allow for population growth.

Even in the early stages of primary health care initiatives, links with secondary and tertiary health services should be established. Those who run the health system, including the medical profession, have a great deal of learning to do before services become reoriented and there is a real willingness to reallocate resources. Mechanisms for referral from the primary health care level to health centres and hospitals need careful attention. So does support to the primary level from the formal services and institutions.

Gaining professional understanding and support are also important. Some countries have systems of compulsory social service by young physicians and nurses, usually in rural areas. Where such systems exist, it should be relatively simple to extend them to primary health care in urban communities. In addition, it is essential from the very start to work at building up support and alliance at high levels in the health administration, in the medical schools, and among political leaders, so that finding resources for the transition from small-scale projects and other successful initiatives to a continuing, comprehensive service is something that is foreseen and aided from the beginning.

The responsibility for comprehensive health care inescapably lies with government agencies. Frequently, nongovernmental organizations are involved—at least initially—in specific local projects. The progress from tiny beginnings to comprehensive coverage will thus raise certain issues concerning relationships between government and nongovernmental organizations, although there will be almost as many problems when nongovernmental organizations are not involved.

From experience reviewed at the Manila consultation, three methods of scaling-up may be identified (Fig. 10). In the first—as, for example, at Olongapo (Philippines) or in the community nursing service in Hong Kong—a project started by a nongovernmental organization is absorbed by the government and becomes an integral part of the public service. The second is a process of cellular multiplication, based on a service model developed and tested on a pilot basis or in a particular local context; any number of new cells could, in theory, be developed and run by nongovernmental organizations. In the third, the government agrees with selected nongovernmental organizations on their roles and functions in the local and national development of urban primary health care, an example being the urban basic services programme in India. These three approaches (and there may be others) are not necessarily mutually exclusive, and the countries and nongovernmental organizations concerned can choose various combinations of them. For example, it may well make sense, once a nongovernmental organization has successfully contributed to primary health care at the local level, for the government to commission it not only to continue the good work locally, but also to undertake broader educational and monitoring activities in support of local services elsewhere.

Another way of looking at scaling-up is shown in Fig. 11. It demonstrates the important point that the process of expansion basically involves learning to fill in the gaps that emerge as the circle grows.

The following major steps need to be taken by governments and nongovernmental organizations to extend useful small-scale projects:

- Evaluate and document the original small-scale experiment.

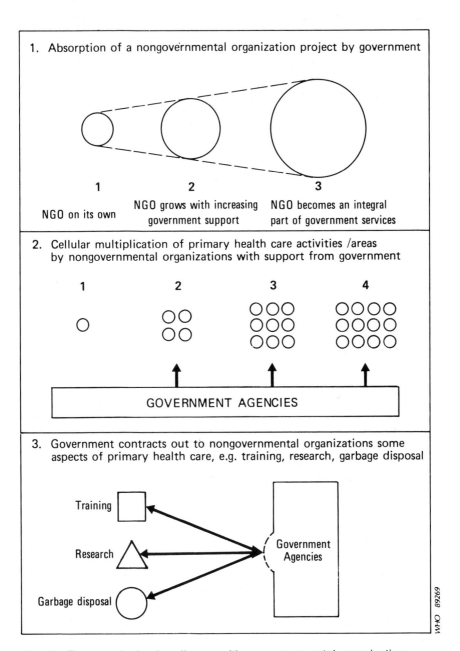

1. Absorption of a nongovernmental organization project by government

1	2	3
NGO on its own	NGO grows with increasing government support	NGO becomes an integral part of government services

2. Cellular multiplication of primary health care activities /areas by nongovernmental organizations with support from government

GOVERNMENT AGENCIES

3. Government contracts out to nongovernmental organizations some aspects of primary health care, e.g. training, research, garbage disposal

Training

Research

Garbage disposal

Government Agencies

WHO 89269

Fig. 10. Three methods of scaling-up with nongovernmental organizations

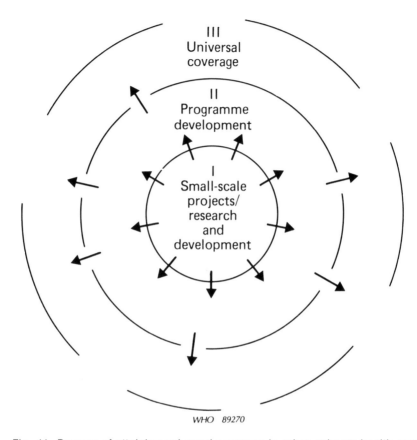

WHO 89270

Fig. 11. Process of attaining universal coverage in urban primary health care

This diagram shows that there are many more things to learn as small-scale projects or research and development projects move up to a second and expanded phase of programme development. Gaps in the middle and outer circles represent issues to be dealt with that could not be anticipated during earlier phases.

- Arrange consultations at the national and provincial levels to discuss the findings and to obtain a commitment from decision-makers at lower than national level to adopt the methodology in their areas.

- Set up experimental projects with different population groups in a wide range of environmental conditions.

- Explain and promote these projects through the mass media.

- At national level, call on the government to allocate additional funds to cover the cost of replication.

For example, programmes in Sri Lanka, after the initial efforts in the capital city of Colombo, and in India, after the initial experiment in Hyderabad, followed the above steps methodically. Today Sri Lanka has extended its programme to all six major cities, and India hopes to involve 200 towns within the next 3 years.

Collaboration between governments and non-governmental organizations

Many voluntary and nongovernmental organizations have developed effective and efficient programmes at low cost, largely owing to flexible management and the commitment and pioneering spirit of their workers. Health authorities can involve such organizations in planning and programme implementation and encourage the coordination of their respective activities, making use of the wealth of experience that many of these organizations possess.

Almost all the countries represented at the Manila consultation had experienced similar difficulties in dealing with nongovernmental organizations at both national and local levels. (The exception was China, which was satisfied with its relationships with nongovernmental organizations.) While assistance from such organizations was regarded as important, and sometimes invaluable, governments often experienced substantial difficulties in incorporating their activities into public policy and planning, and in achieving the necessary coordination. Frequently, liaison and negotiation with nongovernmental organizations add an additional dimension to the burden already placed on scarce management resources. (This applies, for example, in countries where there are overlapping offers of international aid.) Governments may also have difficulty in dealing with the problems regarding resources that often arise in connection with nongovernmental organizations—for example, in deciding whether to take over their funding on a long-term basis or to replicate them.

Sudan provides an interesting example of the complexities of collaboration between governmental and nongovernmental organizations, and has found some constructive ways of tackling the resulting difficulties. At least five international nongovernmental organizations from different countries are heavily involved in urban health care projects in Sudan, together with many Sudanese nongovernmental organizations (women's groups, church groups, and Sudanaid). The major problem of coordinating their activities has been eased by the Government, notably through the secondment of government employees to the main nongovernmental organizations involved; and the holding of joint seminars, workshops, and training courses under the aegis of the Ministry of Health.

151

The governments in Thailand and the Philippines have a flexible relationship with nongovernmental organizations and look to them to undertake new initiatives, particularly in the areas of research and development and community organization. Nongovernmental organizations are considered to be more effective in these areas, because they are not subject to the regulations, procedures, and methods that restrict government agencies. To involve nongovernmental organizations more effectively, government authorities often invite their participation in planning activities and try to reach an agreement on the geographical and sectoral areas they will cover, so that government efforts can be adjusted accordingly. In Thailand, a group of nongovernmental organizations has assisted the Ministry of Health in formulating the list of drugs to be used in primary health care. In Hong Kong, nongovernmental organizations helped to test the community nursing scheme, later incorporated by the Hong Kong Government into the regular health services. In the Philippines, regional coordinating councils are now being created to link the Ministry of Health, various other government offices (chosen on a multisectoral basis), and the relevant nongovernmental organizations.

In China, the primary health care work of the government and various nongovernmental organizations, both local and external, derives its authority from the National Association of Rural Health Workers. The emphasis has traditionally been on activities in the rural areas. Recently, however, several cities in China have started to organize primary health care councils or committees. The relative roles and contributions of governmental and nongovernmental organizations are defined by the requirements of these councils and by neighbourhood, government, and international organizations.

Many specialized agencies of the United Nations, bilateral donor agencies, and international nongovernmental organizations are involved in and support primary health care in urban areas. Their support requires careful coordination within the context of local health needs and priorities, with particular attention to unserved and underserved populations and the urban poor. This can only be achieved by the national authorities, and their aim should be to bring the different types of external assistance together in mutually supportive action for urban development, avoiding overlap and duplication and concentrating on activities that can be continued and expanded with national resources when aid ceases.

At the joint UNICEF/WHO Consultation on Primary Health Care in Urban Areas held in Guayaquil, Ecuador, in 1984, participants outlined the main areas in which progress was needed and feasible:

- *Support.* Support should be based on a joint effort by the organizations and countries concerned. It should take into account the fact that primary health care activities are long-term, so that there must be agreement on plans for their continuation when outside support ends. Activities should emphasize technical cooperation among developing countries and contacts should take place at more than one level of government. Contact at the national level with the international agencies involved is not enough. The participation of municipal —and, in some cases, regional—authorities is vital. Moreover, ministries and departments outside the health sector must be involved. No ministry of health can achieve what is needed in isolation, even with international help.

- *Overall promotion.* International action on urban primary health care is helping to promote public and political awareness of the size and urgency of the health problems of the urban poor. It is important for its momentum to be sustained and indeed increased. One specific suggestion made at the Consultation was that workshops on the subject might be arranged for mayors of large cities. While there is still a need to increase awareness of the gravity of the situation, it is equally important to demonstrate that something worthwhile can be done about it through primary health care

- *Information.* International organizations, such as UNICEF and WHO, have a valuable part to play in the collection, updating, and dissemination of information concerning, for example, demographic trends and morbidity, as well as experience in tackling urban problems. More information is needed on health differentials within cities: such information, collected in any city, could usefully be passed on to others. That applies also to examples of legislation or regulations that promote (or, on the other hand, prejudice) health in urban areas. Case studies would be of great value, as long as they are frank about failures as well as successes and can bring out the lessons to be learnt. Visual and audiovisual material, such as slides, video tapes, and documentary films, can be an excellent means of conveying the setting, the human warmth, and other characteristics of particular projects and programmes. UNICEF and WHO could let people know what is already available and might also, on occasion, develop new material analysing and comparing approaches in different places. The two organizations are also able to clarify and explain the key concepts underlying primary health care, and to provide technical information and advice.

- *Training materials and programmes.* Participants at the Consultation emphasized the importance of training programmes, including the development of appropriate training methods and materials, such as training modules for various categories of professional and nonprofessional staff, including community health workers. Another important need is for management studies. International support could usefully include exchanges of staff between countries, study visits, and similar activities for urban health workers, including health administrators. Apart from their educational value, such visits help to stimulate collaboration between countries with similar problems.

- *Support for primary health care action in countries.* Support for particular primary health care projects and programmes is valuable, not only for launching and sustaining such projects, but for extending the lessons learnt from them to the rest of the health care system. Projects backed by international organizations, such as the World Bank's infrastructure project, can provide useful entry-points for primary health care initiatives in low-income areas. Locally and internationally, therefore, there is a case for seeking out such projects at an early stage and finding the best ways of incorporating a primary health care component. There is also a need for the monitoring and evaluation of initiatives, and for the development of research capabilities in this connection. Special emphasis was placed by the Consultation on the part that UNICEF and WHO might be able to play in helping countries to move from isolated projects towards comprehensive coverage and a corresponding realignment of the whole health care delivery system.

- *Networking.* Networks of communication and mutual support linking all persons and agencies concerned with urban primary health care are especially valuable. It will be useful to develop and extend information networks covering primary health care workers and managers, city administrators and government departments (not only those directly concerned with health), universities, the media, nongovernmental organizations, and a wide range of international agencies.

Collaboration between cities

Many international meetings have been held in the past few years on the problems of health and urban development. These have served a useful purpose by facilitating exchanges of experience and

154

arousing official and public concern over the urgent need for effective action to improve the general condition of the urban poor.

However, a stage has now been reached at which it may be more useful to promote a form of direct collaboration between cities, so that those with common problems can share experiences and ideas and together can consider, in depth, the advantages of various possible approaches.

This collaboration might be organized mainly on a regional basis because of the similarity of conditions within a region. Alternatively, exchanges between cities with comparable problems, but in completely different cultural or geographical settings, might provide a greater stimulus to innovation.

The type of collaboration envisaged need not be limited to capital or major cities but might usefully be encouraged between cities of the second or third rank facing the problems of rapid urbanization, but not yet totally overwhelmed by them.

The conventional type of international meeting could continue, but more frequent direct consultations between two or more cities with similar interests would probably be more useful, as well as being fully consistent with the concept of technical cooperation between developing countries.

The conclusions and content of these consultations would be of interest to people in other cities contemplating extending primary health care coverage. In recent years, reports on the introduction of primary health care in urban areas have, naturally enough, dealt mainly with plans, targets, and inputs. After some years of operation, however, it is important, whenever possible, to lay stress on evaluation and on the actual impact on health of the measures employed.

Collaboration between cities should obviously include exchanges of data on health variations within them, as well as examples of legislation or regulations that have promoted or prejudiced the health of the urban poor. Honest case studies are of great value.

The involvement of national staff at many different levels in a programme of collaboration between cities should foster the development of informal links between all those concerned.

Chapter 6

Conclusions

During the coming two decades, one of the most important development trends in the world will be the rapid growth in the number of people living in cities, especially in the developing countries. The growth rate for the urban population is far higher than for the population outside the cities. This increase will further aggravate major health issues in urban and periurban settings, particularly where low-income groups of the population live. The root cause of the urban crisis is poverty. Poverty in rural areas drives people to the cities; urban poverty keeps them in slums and squatter settlements with all the associated major risks to health.

Urban health problems are complex and linked with socioeconomic and developmental issues. Levels of income, water supply, food and nutrition, housing, sanitation, environmental pollution and safety, education, and facilities, all have an obvious impact on health. To improve the health of the unserved and underserved people in urban areas, the health sectors need intensive and coordinated support and increased developmental action from the health-related sectors. To initiate this coordinated action, strong political will and commitment are paramount.

The existing information is not sufficient to permit assessment of the health situation and the health-related issues of the urban poor. At present, most of the available information is in the form of aggregated urban data and city averages. There is a great need to identify the basic issues affecting the health of the urban poor and for information to be oriented towards stratified planning for urban health. Health care delivery systems and services accordingly need to be reoriented to these needs. Cooperation within health systems and partnership with other interested parties, particularly private and nongovernmental organizations, should be encouraged.

Despite these complexities, some countries have undertaken action and learned valuable lessons which need to be shared. Most people—including most professional health workers—do not yet recognize how serious the health problems of the urban poor are; still less how desperate they may become. Once the problems are recognized, there can be no acceptable excuse for inaction.

The basic features of an appropriate strategy for tackling the health problems of the urban poor should be clear from this book. They may be summarized as follows:

- Do simple, inexpensive things with a proven impact.

- Take intersectoral action, rather than concentrating on medical care services.

- Involve people in their own health and treatment, and take into account their judgements about priorities.

- Do not settle for action on a small, experimental scale, while ignoring how widespread the problems of urban poverty and ill health actually are.

- Work towards a national pattern of health care that will deal with the problems in question on a wide front, taking into account cities across the nation and concentrating on their poorest inhabitants.

A dozen or so human problems can lay claim to be the most serious of our time. Among them is the predicament of the urban poor in the poorest countries of the world. Their position is as appalling as their courage is impressive. To help them does not require new knowledge so much as a change of approach from the rest of us.

What is more, the lessons thereby learnt are likely to be relevant elsewhere. Health for all depends not only on professional skills, but on personal ability, a healthy environment, and sensible choices in the use of scarce resources. The poor urban communities are showing us the road we need to take.

References

1. WHO/UNICEF. *Primary health care. Report of the International Conference on Primary Health Care, Alma-Ata.* Geneva, World Health Organization, 1978. (Health for All Series, No. 1), p. 23.

2. *Global Strategy for Health for All by the Year 2000.* Geneva, World Health Organization, 1981 (Health for All Series, No. 3).

3. ROSSI-ESPAGNET, A. Health and the urban poor. *World health,* July 1983.

4. STOTT, G. & TABIBZADEH, I. *Attaining universal coverage by primary health care in urban areas.* Unpublished document prepared at the WHO/UNICEF Interregional Consultation on Primary Health Care in Urban Areas, Manila, Philippines, 7–11 July 1986. (A limited number of copies are available from the Division of Strengthening of Health Services, World Health Organization, Geneva, Switzerland).

5. UNITED NATIONS FUND FOR POPULATION ACTIVITIES. *Report of the International Conference on Population and the Urban Future, Rome, 1–4 September 1980.* New York.

6. UNITED NATIONS FUND FOR POPULATION ACTIVITIES. Rome Declaration on Population and the Urban Future. *International Conference on Population and the Urban Future, Rome, 1–4 September 1980.* New York.

7. UNITED NATIONS. *The prospect of world urbanization* (revised 1984, 1985). New York, 1987 (Population Studies, No. 101; ST/ESA/SER.A/101).

8. UNITED NATIONS. *Urbanization and components of urban and city population growth.* New York, 1983 (document IESA/P/ICP.1984/EG.11/23, prepared for the International Conference on Population, Mexico City, 1984).

9. TELLER, C. H. *The population dynamics of urbanization and some implications for the health sector.* Paper prepared for the PAHO/AMRO Regional Technical Consultation on the Development of Health Services and Primary Health Care in Urban Areas and Big Cities, Washington, DC, 16–20 November 1981.

10. UNITED NATIONS. *Migration, population growth and employment in metropolitan areas of selected developing countries.* New York, 1985 (document ST/ESA/SER.R57).

11. ORGANIZATION FOR ECONOMIC COOPERATION AND DEVELOPMENT. *Managing urban change. Vol. 1. Policies and finance.* Paris, 1983.

12. HIRSCHMAN, C. Recent urbanization trends in peninsular Malaysia. *Demography*, **13**(4): 445–461 (1976).

13. UNITED NATIONS. *Role and potential of technical cooperation among developing countries in rural–urban migration and economic development.* New York, 1981 (document TCDC/2/10).

14. UNITED NATIONS EDUCATIONAL, SCIENTIFIC AND CULTURAL ORGANIZATION. *Fourth world and human rights.* Paris, 1980.

15. FERNAND-LAURENT, J. Introduction. In: *Human rights in urban areas.* Paris, United Nations Educational, Scientific and Cultural Organization, 1983, pp. 9–10.

16. WRENSKI, J. The poorest of the poor in the city: age-old drive for human rights. In: *Human rights in urban areas.* Paris, United Nations Educational, Scientific and Cultural Organization, 1983, pp. 22–28.

17. WOLF, S. *Concepts and measurements of poverty.* Geneva, United Nations Research Institute for Social Development, 1981.

18. MUNCIE, P. Task force defines strategy to alleviate urban poverty. *Finance and development*, **13**: 2 (1976).

19. HOLMES, T. H. & RAHE, R. H. The social readjustment rating scale. *Journal of psychosomatic research*, **11**: 213–218 (1967).

20. INTERNATIONAL LABOUR OFFICE. *Child labour and health. Proceedings of the First International Workshop, Nairobi, Kenya, 2–3 December 1982.*

21. LEVIN, L. Too young to work. *World health*, January–February 1984, pp. 24–27.

22. LEVIN, L. Child labour: stocktaking. *International children's rights monitor*, **1**(1): 10–13 (1983).

23. SWEPSTON, L. Child labour. Its regulation by ILO standards and national legislation. *International labour review*, **121**(5): 577–593 (1982).

24. SHAH, P. M. Health status of working and street children and alternative approaches to their health care. In: *Advances in international maternal and child health*, Vol. 7. Clarendon Press, Oxford, 1987, pp. 70–93.

25. The sexual exploitation of children. *International children's rights monitor*, **1**(1): 6–7 (1983).

26. Child abuse: the ultimate betrayal. *Time*, 5 September 1983, pp. 30–32.

27. GENTILINI, M. ET AL. Urbanisme et santé publique sous les tropiques. *Bulletin de la Société de Pathologie exotique et de ses filiales*, **76**(3): 276–284 (1983).

28. PUFFER, R. R. & GRIFFITH, G. W. *Patterns of urban mortality.* Washington, DC, Pan American Health Organization, 1967 (Scientific Publication No. 151).

29. KHANJANASTHITI, P. & WRAY, J. D. Early protein-calorie malnutrition in slum areas of Bangkok municipality, 1970–1971. *Journal of the Medical Association of Thailand*, **57**(7): 357–366 (1974).

30. ROHDE, J. E. Why the other half dies: the science and politics of child mortality in the Third World. *Assignment children*, **61–62**: 35–67 (1983).

31. COULIBALY, N. Place et approches des problèmes de la tuberculose à Abidjan. *Médecine d'Afrique noire*, **28**: 447–449 (July 1981)

32. BENYOUSSEF, A. ET AL. Santé, migration et urbanization: une étude collective au Sénégal. *Bulletin of the World Health Organization*, **49**: 517–537 (1973).

33. KEREJAN, H. & N'DA KONAN. Approche des problèmes alimentaires et nutritionnels d'une mégalopolis africaine. *Médecine d'Afrique noire*, **28**(7): 479–482 (1981).

34. VINOCUR, P. Clasificación funcional de poblaciones desnutridas en Costa Rica. *Boletín informativo de SIN*, **2**(1) (1980).

35. VALVERDE, V. & COLL, M. *Clasificación funcional de problemas nutricionales en El Salvador*. Guatemala, Ministry of Public Health and Social Welfare of El Salvador and the Nutrition Institute of Central America and Panama (IN-CAP), 1977.

36. General Secretariat of the National Economic Planning Board and the Nutrition Institute of Central America and Panama (INCAP). *Final report of the study on "Regionalisación de problemas nutricionales en Guatemala"*. Guatemala, 1980 (unpublished document).

37. PRASADA RAO, T. M. ET AL. Nutritional status of children in urban slums around Hyderabad City. *Indian journal of medical research*, **62**(10): 1492–1498 (1974).

38. PARAMITA SUDHARTO. Experiences in the field of urban primary health care in Jakarta. In: *Report of UNICEF/WHO Meeting on Primary Health Care in Urban Areas, Geneva, July 1983*. Unpublished WHO document SHS/HSR/83.1.[1]

39. BRINK, E. W. ET AL. The Egyptian National Nutrition Survey, 1978. *Bulletin of the World Health Organization*, **61**(5): 853–860 (1983).

40. SHUBERT, C. *Reflections on primary health projects among the urban poor: implications for large-scale programme development*. Paper presented at the UNICEF/WHO Interregional Consultation on Primary Health Care in Urban Areas, Manila Philippines, 7–11 July 1986. Unpublished WHO document SHS/IHS/86.1.[1]

41. BASTA, S. S. Nutrition and health in low income areas of the Third World. *Ecology of food and nutrition*, **6**: 113–124 (1977).

42. *Encuesta de hogares*. Ministry of Health, Colombia, 1970.

43. WORLD HEALTH ORGANIZATION. *Development of indicators for monitoring progress towards health for all by the year 2000*. Geneva, 1981 (Health for All Series, No. 4).

---

[1] A limited number of copies are available from: Division of Strengthening of Health Services, World Health Organization, 1211 Geneva 27, Switzerland.

44. WORLD HEALTH ORGANIZATION. *Health programme evaluation.* Geneva, 1981 (Health for All Series, No. 6).

45. CULYER, A. J. *Health indicators: an international study for the European Science Foundation.* Worcester, Billing & Sons, 1983.

46. *Minimum evaluation procedures for water supply and sanitation projects.* Unpublished WHO document ETS/83.1, CDD/OPR/83.1, 1983. (A limited number of copies are available from Diarrhoeal Diseases Control, World Health Organization, 1211 Geneva 27, Switzerland.)

47. *Report of the UNICEF/WHO Meeting on Primary Health Care in Urban Areas, Geneva, 25–29 July 1983.* Unpublished WHO document SHS/HSR/83.1.[1]

48. OLUDAYISI ODUNTAN, S. *The health of Nigerian children of school age (six to fifteen years): a thesis.* Unpublished WHO document, APR/MCH/68. (A limited number of copies are available from Maternal and Child Health, World Health Organization, 1211 Geneva 27, Switzerland.)

49. MINISTRY OF HEALTH AND WELFARE. Department of Public Health of Mexico City. *Plan for primary health care in peri-urban areas: summary 1977.*

50. HARDIE, M. & MORRIS, R. Patchwork in big cities, *Lancet*, 1: 287 (1982).

51. Primary health care in slum areas of Guayaquil, Ecuador. *Assignment children,* 63/64: 115–131 (1983).

52. BERTRAND, W. E. & LEVINE, A. A rapid survey technique for "appropriate technology" indicators in developing urban areas. *Social indicators research,* 7: 237–249 (1980).

53. BERTRAND, W. E. ET AL. A methodology for determining high-risk components in rural environments. *International journal of epidemiology,* 8(2): 161–166 (1979).

54. HASSOUNA, W. A. Executive summary of the health service assessment study. *The health service researcher,* 3: 1–30 (1982).

55. ROSENBLATT, R. Journalism and the larger truth. *Time,* 2 July 1984.

56. BRIDGERS, W. F. A brief chapter in the politics of prevention research. *Journal of public health policy,* 5(1): 5–91 (1984).

57. WHO Technical Report Series, No. 694, 1983 (*Research for the reorientation of national health systems:* report of a WHO Study Group).

58. TAYLOR, C. E. *The uses of health systems research.* Geneva, World Health Organization, 1984 (Public Health Papers, No. 78).

59. *UNICEF/WHO Inter-regional Consultation on Primary Health Care in Urban Areas, Manila, Philippines, 7–11 July 1986.* Unpublished WHO document, SHS/IHS/86.1.[1]

60. Training: A high-return investment. *The urban edge,* 8(3), March/April 1984.

---

[1] A limited number of copies are available from: Division of Strengthening of Health services, World Health Organization, 1211 Geneva 27, Switzerland.

61. *Strengthening ministries of health for primary health care*. Geneva, World Health Organization, 1984 (WHO Offset Publication No. 82).

62. *The role of hospitals in primary health care: a report of a conference sponsored by the Aga Khan Foundation and the World Health Organization, 22–26 November 1981, Karachi, Pakistan*. Geneva, Aga Khan Foundation/WHO, 1981.

63. WHO Technical Report Series, No. 744, 1987 (*Hospitals and health for all: report of a WHO Expert Committee on the Role of Hospitals at the First Referral Level*).

64. PAINE, L. H. W & SIEM TJAM, F. *Hospitals and the health care revolution*. Geneva, World Health Organization, 1988.

65. *Primary health care—the Chinese experience*. Geneva, World Health Organization, 1983.

66. OAKLEY, P. *Community involvement in health development: an examination of the critical issues*. Geneva, World Health Organization 1989.

67. UNITED NATIONS. *Urban slums and squatter settlements in the third world. Note by the Secretary-General* (paper prepared for the Regional Preparatory Conference for Habitat, United Nations Conference on Human Settlements). New York, 1975 (document A/CONF.70/RPC/9).

68. UNITED NATIONS ECONOMIC AND SOCIAL COUNCIL. *Urban basic services reaching children and women of the urban poor*. Report by the Executive Director. New York, 1982 (document E/ICEF/L.1440).

69. JOHNSTON, M. The labyrinth of community participation: experiences from Indonesia. *Community development journal*, 17(3): 202–207 (1982).

70. HOLLENSTEINER, M. R. People power: community participation in the planning of human settlements. *Assignment children*, **40**: 11–47 (1977).

71. UNITED NATIONS ECONOMIC AND SOCIAL COUNCIL. *Urban basic services: reaching children and women of the urban poor. Addendum; a summary of nine case studies*. New York, 1982, unpublished document E/ICEF/L.1440/Add.1.

72. RAM, E. R. & VASANT, M. E. A community kitchen in the Kamanves slum, India. *Assignment children*, **43**: 47–56 (1978).

73. BARBEDETTE, L. Animation d'une zone d'extension spontanée de Douala, Cameroun, *Assignment children*, **43**: 63–92 (1978).

74. HOLLENSTEINER, M. R. Government strategies for urban areas and community participation. *Assignment children*, **57/58**: 43–64 (1982).

75. WHO Technical Report Series, No. 780, 1989 (*Strengthening the performance of community health workers in primary health care*: report of a WHO Study Group).

76. MCKEOWN, T. *The role of medicine: dream, mirage or nemesis*, 2nd ed. Oxford, Blackwell, 1979.

77. MCKINLEY, J. B. & MCKINLEY, S. M. The questionable contributions of medical measures to the decline of mortality in the United States in the twentieth century. *Milbank Memorial Fund quarterly (health and society)*, 55(3): 405–428 (1977).

78. VOHRA, N. N. Better health in Delhi's slums. *World health,* July 1983, pp. 22–24.

79. SIVARAMAKRISHNAN, K. C. Towards better metropolitan management: the management of Asian cities. *The urban edge,* **6**(10), November 1982.

80. SIVARAMAKRISHNAN, K. C. *Indian urban scene 1978.* (Document available from the Registrar, Indian Institute of Advanced Study, Pashthanati, Vivas, Simla, India.)

81. *NADI programme: a joint effort between the people and the Government to improve the quality of urban life.* Kuala Lumpur, Ministry of Federal Territory, 1980 (unpublished document).

82. The Metropolitan Manila Management Conference. *The urban edge,* **6**(10), November 1982.

83. PUFFER, R. R. & SERRANO, C. V. *Patterns of mortality in childhood: report of the Inter-American Investigation of Mortality in Childhood.* Washington, DC, Pan American Health Organization, 1973 (PAHO Scientific Publication, No. 262).

84. DATTA BANIK, N. D. Some observations on feeding programmes, nutrition and growth of preschool children in an urban community. *Indian journal of pediatrics,* **44**: 139–149 (1977).

85. DATTA BANIK, N. D. Feeding habits and weaning practices in infants and preschool children in slum areas in New Delhi. *Archives of child health,* **21**(3): 51–57 (1979).

86. DELA LUZ ALBAREX, M. ET AL. Características de familias urbanas con lactante desnutrido. *Archivos latinoamericanos de nutrición,* **29** (2): 220–232 (1979).

87. SIGULEM, D. M. & TUDISCO, E. S. Aleitamento natural em diferentes classes de renda no municipio de São Paulo. *Archivos latinoamericanos de nutrición,* **30**(3): 400–416 (1980).

88. MINISTRY OF PUBLIC HEALTH OF MOROCCO. Enquête national sur l'état de nutrition des enfants de moins de 4 ans. *Bulletin de la santé publique,* New Series **3** (54) (1973).

89. NELSON, J. & MANDL, P. E. Peri-urban malnutrition, a neglected problem. *Assignment children,* **43**: 25 (1978).

90. JELLIFFE, E. F. P. The impact of the food industry on the nutritional status of infants and preschool children in developing countries. In: *Priorities in child nutrition in developing countries,* Vol. 2, Cambridge, MA, Harvard University School of Public Health, 1975.

91. YEH, S. Urban low-income housing in South-East Asia. In: Richards, P. J. & Thomson, A. M., ed., *Basic needs and the urban poor.* London, Croom Helm, 1984.

92. *Health principles of housing.* Geneva, World Health Organization, 1989.

93. *Improving environmental health conditions in low-income settlements: a community-based approach to identifying needs and priorities.* Geneva, World Health Organization, 1987 (WHO Offset Publication, No. 100).

94. *Environmental health in rural and urban development and housing.* Unpublished WHO document EPF/RUD/84.1.[1]

95. INTERNATIONAL DRINKING WATER SUPPLY AND SANITATION DECADE. *Review of mid-decade progress (as at December 1985).* Unpublished WHO document, 1987.[1]

96. ISMARTONO, Y. It's the government's job to collect the garbage. *UNICEF news,* No. 15: 12–14 (1983).

97. *Global review of human settlements.* New York, United Nations Centre for Human Settlements (HABITAT), 1976 (document A/CONF.70/A31), p. 121.

98. *World housing survey 1974: an overview of the state of housing, building and planning within human settlements.* New York, United Nations, 1976 (document ST/ESA/30).

99. MORELL, S. & MORELL, D. *Six slums in Bangkok.* Bangkok, United Nations Children's Fund, 1972.

100. WHITE, M. B. & WHITE, H. D. *The power of the people: community action in Korea.* Urban Industrial Mission, East Asian Christian Conference, 1973.

101. DE GEYNAT, W. Atención primaria de salud en zonas urbanas y rurales de los países en desarrollo: semejanzas y diferencias. *Boletín de la Oficina Sanitaria Panamericana,* **94**(5): 441–460 (1983).

102. UNITED NATIONS CHILDREN'S FUND. *State of the world's children.* New York, 1986.

103. INTERNATIONAL DRINKING WATER SUPPLY AND SANITATION DECADE, 1981–1990. *Global sector concepts for water supply and sanitation, March 1987* (prepared under the international cooperation programme between the World Health Organization and the German Federal Ministry for Economic Cooperation). Unpublished WHO document, 1987.[1]

104. *Intersectoral action for health. The role of intersectoral cooperation in national strategies for health for all.* Geneva, World Health Organization 1986.

105. ANKER, R. An analysis of fertility differentials in developing countries. *Review of economics and statistics,* **60**(1): 58–69 (1978).

106. *Education.* Washington, DC, World Bank, 1974 (Sector working paper).

107. *Health.* Washington, DC, World Bank, 1974 (Sector policy paper).

108. BOULIER, B. L. Population policy and income distribution, In: Frank, C. R. & Webb, R. C., ed. *Income distribution and growth in the less developed countries.* Washington, DC, Brooking Institution.

109. YUSOF, K. "Sang Kancil"—care for urban squatters in Malaysia. *World health forum,* **3**(3): 278–281 (1982).

110. DIAZ, R. Restructuring services to reach the urban poor in Kuala Lumpur. *Assignment children,* **57–58**: 135–136 (1982).

---

[1] A limited number of copies are available from: Division of Environmental Health, World Health Organization, 1211 Geneva 27, Switzerland.

111. HERRERA DAVILA, J. *Atención integral al niño y su familia en los pueblos jovenes del zono sur de Lima Metropolitana.* Paper presented at the International Seminar/Workshop on Urban Primary Health Care, Popayan, Colombia, 5–9 July 1982.

112. WORLD HEALTH ORGANIZATION. *National decision-making for primary health care. A study by the UNICEF/WHO Joint Committee on Health Policy.* Geneva, 1981.

113 *Report of the International Meeting on Strengthening District Health Systems Based on Primary Health Care, Harare, Zimbabwe, 3–7 August 1987.* Unpublished WHO document SHS/DHS/87.13, Rev. 1.[1]

114 WHO Technical Report Series, No. 766, 1988 (*Strengthening ministries of health for primary health care*: report of a WHO Expert Committee).

115. *Joint UNICEF/WHO Consultation on Primary Health Care in Urban Areas, Guayaquil, Ecuador.* Unpublished WHO document SHS/84.5, 1984.[1]

---

[1] A limited number of copies are available from: Division of Strengthening of Health Services, World Health Organization, 1211 Geneva 27, Switzerland.

Annex

Indicators of social development in Thailand

In Bangkok, Thailand, the authorities have recently introduced a "basic minimum needs" community survey and information system. This is intended to measure 33 indicators of overall development and to compare them with target levels. Thus, the system provides baseline information for individual households and for the community, and identifies the specific households and sectors where improvement is needed. Table A1 provides details on the indicators and gives the targets to be achieved by the year 2000, while Fig. A1 indicates the main components in the process by which the strategy is to be applied.

Table AI. Basic minimum needs and targets to be achieved by the year 2000 in Bangkok

Basic minimum needs	Breakdown of needs	Indicators	Targets	1986-1991	1992-1997	by 2001
1. People consume hygienic foods in sufficient amounts according to their bodily needs	1.1. Infants and preschool children (0–6 years) are under nutritional surveillance and do not suffer from malnutrition to an extent harmful to their health	Standard weights and heights for age	Proportion of children with first-(1), second-(2), and third-degree (3) malnutrition should be:	(1) not more than 30% (2) not more than 5% (3) nil	not more than 20% nil nil	not more than 10% nil nil
	1.2. Schoolchildren (7–14 years) receive enough nourishing food for their bodily needs	Standard weights and heights for age	Proportion of children weighing lower than the standard should not exceed:	10%	7%	5%
	1.3 Pregnant women consume sufficient amounts of food	Newborns weigh not less than 3000 g	Proportion of newborns having a birth-weight of 3000 g or over should be:	70%	80%	90%
	1.4 Families consume hygienic food	Absence of acute diarrhoea.	Annual morbidity from acute diarrhoea should not exceed:	15%	8%	5%
2. People have appropriate housing and a sanitary environment	2.1 Houses are made of appropriate and durable materials	Houses are made of appropriate and durable materials and built to last at least five years	Proportion of houses having durable roofing and walls should be not less than:	70%	80%	90%
	2.2 Families have sanitary arrangements in their houses	Clean houses with collection places for garbage and animal waste and waste-water drainage	Proportion of families with sanitary household arrangements should be not less than:	70%	80%	90%

Table A1. (*continued*)

Basic minimum needs	Breakdown of needs	Indicators	Targets	1986–1991	1992–1997	by 2001
	2.3 Families have sanitary latrines	Houses with water-sealed latrines	Proportion of families having water-sealed latrines should be not less than:	70%	80%	90%
	2.4 Families have adequate supplies of clean drinking-water (rain-water, filtered water, piped water, sanitary well-water).	Sufficient quantity of clean drinking-water available	Proportion of families having sufficient clean drinking-water should be not less than:	70%	80%	90%
3. People have access to the basic social services needed in their daily lives and occupations	3.1 Children and young people have access to basic services	(*a*) By 1 year of age, children are fully immunized against tuberculosis, diphtheria, pertussis, poliomyelitis, and measles	(*a*) Proportion of children under 1 year receiving full immunization should not be less than:	70%	85%	95%
		(*b*) Children aged 4–6 years receive booster immunization against diphtheria, pertussis, tetanus, and poliomyelitis (twice)	(*b*) Proportion of pre-school children (4–6 years) receiving full booster immunization should be:	70%	85%	95%
		(*c*) Children are taken care of by families	(*c*) Proportion of pre-school children (under 7 years) receiving proper care from families should be:	80%	90%	100%
		(*d*) Children receive compulsory education	(*d*) Number of school-age children (7–14+ years) receiving education should be:	80%	95%	100%

3.2 People have access to basic social and occupational services	(a) People receive news and information relating to occupation, nutrition, health, hygiene and prevention of public disasters (b) People have opportunities for regular recreation and exercise	(a) Number of families receiving news and information relating to occupation, hygiene, and prevention of public disasters should be: (b) Each community should have a place where the people can go for recreation:	60% 1 place	70% 1 place	80% 1 place
	(c) Pregnant women have at least 4 visits for antenatal care (d) Disabled persons and disaster victims receive proper services (e) People aged 14–50 years are literate	(c) Proportion of pregnant women having at least 4 visits for antenatal care: (d) Proportion of occupationally disabled persons receiving help: (e) The literacy rate among people aged 14–50 years is:	70% 70% 100%	80% 80% 100%	90% 90% 100%

Table A1. (continued)

Basic minimum needs	Breakdown of needs	Indicators	Targets	1986–1991	1992–1997	by 2001
4. People's lives and property are fully protected	4.1 People are protected against crime	Security measures are effective	The frequency of severe crime cases (rape, robbery, arson, crimes causing severe injury or death) should not exceed:	6 cases a year; there should be a guard system	4 cases a year; there should be a guard system	2 cases a year; there should be a guard system
	4.2 People can prevent public disasters and provide disaster relief services	(a) There is a system for preventing public disaster (b) The people themselves can prevent and suppress public disasters	(a) and (b) The community should have a fire prevention system, and the number of chemical fire extinguishers should be:	10 per community	15 per community	20 chemical extinguishers and 6 engine extinguishers per community
5. People can produce or acquire sufficient food to live on	5.1 People farm, using proper agricultural techniques	Everyone can farm, using proper agricultural techniques	Proportion of farming families using proper agricultural techniques should be at least:	80%, with 70% having profitable returnsable returns	90%, with 80% having profitable returnsable returns	95%, with 90% having profitable returns
	5.2 People can acquire enough food to eat	People have enough food for 3 meals a day	Proportion of families having 3 meals a day should be:	70%	80%	90%

6. Families can control the spacing and number of children as they wish	6.1 Families practise family planning.			
	(a) Proportion of couples having no more than 2 children should be not less than:	50%	60%	80%
	(b) Proportion of couples spacing pregnancies at least 2 years apart should be not less than:	50%	60%	80%
	(c) Proportion of couples using family planning techniques should be not less than:	70%	80%	90%
7. People participate in developing their lives and in determining their future	7.1 People participate in developing the economic, social, cultural, and environmental aspects of their lives			
	(a) Number of people exercising their voting rights in the election of the community development committee should be not less than:	60%	70%	80%
	(b) There are organized efforts to set up social and economic development groups in each community	1 social and 1 economic development group	1 social and 1 economic development group	1 social and 1 economic development group
	(c) There are organized efforts to set up a group to safeguard public property	1 group for each type of property	1 group for each type of property	1 group for each type of property
	(d) Proportion of families participating in traditional activities should be not less than:	40%	50%	60%

Table A1. (continued)

Basic minimum needs	Breakdown of needs	Indicators	Targets	1986–1991	1992–1997	by 2001
	7.2 People participate in the process of determining their future	(a) People exercise their voting rights in the election of representatives at every level on the democratic pattern	(a) Proportion of people exercising their voting rights at an election should be not less than:	50%	60%	70%
		(b) The community organization established to develop the community can draw up and implement the necessary plan, monitor progress, and maintain the work by themselves: this means specifically that there should be a committee meeting at least 6 times a year; that it should have written details of the plan, the problem-solving activities involved, and the persons responsible; and that it should mobilize all local resources to solve the relevant problems in accordance with the plan	(b) Community participation in an organization to draw up and implement a plan for community development, and to monitor progress and maintain the work by themselves is:	100%	100%	100%

8. People have better morale	8.1 People lead their lives according to their religious creed	(a) People do not drink alcohol, gamble, or abuse drugs	(a) Number of people not drinking alcohol, gambling, or abusing drugs:	100%	100%	100%
		(b) People participate in activities to commemorate important religious days or events	(b) Number of families participating in activities to commemorate important religious days or events:	50%	60%	70%
	8.2 People adopt the basic social values	People do not overspend on either religious or traditional acitivities	Number of families not overspending on either religious or traditional activities:	60%	70%	80%

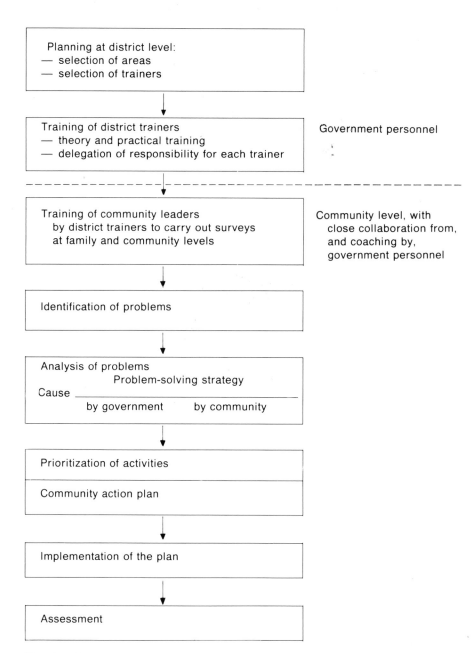

Fig. A1. Process for the application of the basic minimum needs strategy in the development of congested communities in the Bangkok metropolis